CONTENTS

Preface to the third edition

With the exception of editors' families—who always check that they have received due credit for their suffering—hardly anyone reads the Preface to a medical textbook. Nevertheless, we hope that the rest of this book will be heavily thumbed, and there is therefore a chance that it will fall open at this page. If so, please read on!

It is only four years since the last edition of the *Handbook of Diabetes* came out, so does this third edition add anything? We believe so. Firstly, there have been substantial advances in the field of diabetes, as well as some lost ground and a few tactical retreats. On the therapeutic front, various new treatments—glitazones, glitinides, phosphodiesterase inhibitors, long-acting insulin analogues—are now establishing themselves in routine clinical practice. Meanwhile, possible new pathogenic mechanisms, such as inflammatory mediators in type 2 diabetes, are being explored and tested. Also, the hard evidence that hyperglycaemia and raised blood pressure play crucial roles in diabetic tissue complications is at last being exploited to improve the everyday management of the disease. Sadly, the world has moved on for diabetes, as it has for many other things that we would prefer to be without. Twenty-first century civilization is going pear-shaped (or, more accurately, apple-shaped) and, feeding off the pandemic of obesity, type 2 diabetes is on the rampage throughout the world. Most depressing of all is the appearance of type 2 diabetes in childhood and adolescence; the label of 'maturity-onset', now naïve as well as dubious, must finally be laid to rest forever.

This new edition shares with its predecessors our intention to provide an easy-to-read, up-to-date and well-illustrated précis of the most important aspects of the science and clinical practice of diabetes. Both previous editions of the *Handbook* were warmly received, and this has given us great pleasure. Our readership has spanned a wide range of health-care professionals, including doctors (young and old, specialist and generalist, within and outside hospitals), diabetes specialist nurses, dieticians, podiatrists and students of medicine as well as its allied professions and the basic sciences. We are also delighted that the *Handbook* has proved a useful source of information for people with diabetes. If this edition succeeds in making diabetes interesting, exciting and widely comprehensible, then our main ambitions will have been met.

As always, we have many friends and colleagues to thank, and nobody to blame but ourselves. For us, these books present a wonderful opportunity to gather wisdom from the top scientists and practitioners in diabetes from around the world. We are immensely grateful to all 130 contributors to the third edition of the *Textbook of Diabetes*, who have generously allowed us to distil their work into this *Handbook*. Two-thirds of the current contributors were new, and have provided fresh authority and insights into many challenging problems. Putting this edition beside its two predecessors gives a dramatic illustration of the evolution of book design over the last fifteen years—a process in which Blackwell Publishing have been world leaders. Our particular thanks go to our Commissioning Editor, Alison Brown, and to Claire Bonnett (our Editorial Assistant), Nick Morgan (Senior Production Editor), and all the members of their team. The Designers' Collective masterminded another fabulous design which, once again, sets the *Handbook* head and shoulders above most medical texts. Finally, we are indebted to our families who have, as always, given us their selfless support and far more encouragement than we deserve. To them, our heartfelt thanks, even though we still don't quite understand why they keep letting us do this.

GARETH WILLIAMS
JOHN C. PICKUP
Bristol & London, January 2004

INTRODUCTION TO DIABETES

HANDBOOK OF DIABETES 3RD EDITION

Diabetes mellitus is a condition in which there is a chronically raised blood glucose concentration. It is caused by an absolute or relative lack of the hormone insulin – that is, insulin is not being produced by the pancreas, or there is insufficient insulin or insulin action for the body's needs.

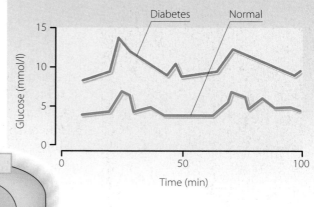

FIGURE 1.1
Raised blood glucose concentrations in diabetes.

Impaired insulin secretion

- β-cell destruction: type 1 diabetes
- Impaired β-cell function: type 2 diabetes

β cell

↓ Insulin

Insulin resistance

- Type 2 diabetes

↓ Biological effects

Target tissues

FIGURE 1.2
Defects in islet β cell and in insulin action in type 1 and 2 diabetes.

The two main types of diabetes are 'type 1' (formerly called insulin-dependent) and 'type 2' (formerly called noninsulin-dependent) diabetes. Type 1 diabetes presents mainly in childhood and early adult life and accounts for about 15% of cases of diabetes in Europe and North America. It is caused by an autoimmune destruction of the insulin-producing β cells of the islets of Langerhans in the pancreas, resulting in absolute insulin deficiency.

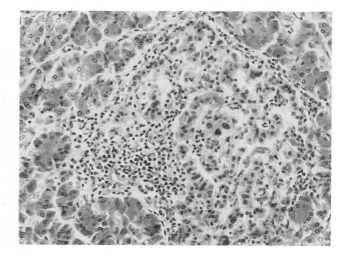

FIGURE 1.3
Inflammatory cells within the islet in type 1 diabetes, associated with autoimmune destruction of the β cells.

third edition

Handbook of
Diabetes

To Caroline, Timothy, Joanna, Sally and Pippa;
and Selma, Matthew, Charlotte and Joshua

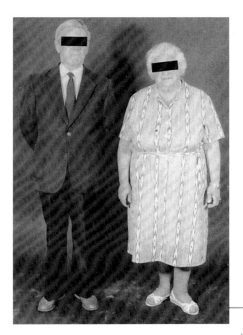

Type 2 diabetes is usually a disease of the middle-aged or elderly. It is the most common type of diabetes, representing about 85% of cases in most Caucasian populations and Western countries, but more than 95% of diabetes in developing countries. It is caused by both impaired insulin secretion and 'resistance' to the action of insulin at its target cells. About 80% of type 2 diabetic patients are obese – obesity and underactivity are major risk factors for developing this type of diabetes. Type 2 diabetes is now becoming a problem in children, with an increasing frequency in many countries that is paralleled by the increase in childhood obesity.

FIGURE 1.4
Lean and obese patients with type 2 diabetes.

One of the most important clinical features of all forms of diabetes is its association with serious tissue complications. These generally occur after several years of diabetes and affect the small blood vessels (microangiopathy) in the eye, kidney and nerves. *Diabetic retinopathy* is the most common cause of blindness in the working-age group in the Western world. *Diabetic nephropathy* is a major cause of kidney failure, while peripheral and autonomic *neuropathy* can contribute to foot ulcers, impotence, diarrhoea, postural hypotension and other disorders. There is good evidence that diabetic microangiopathy, at least, is related to the duration and severity of hyperglycaemia.

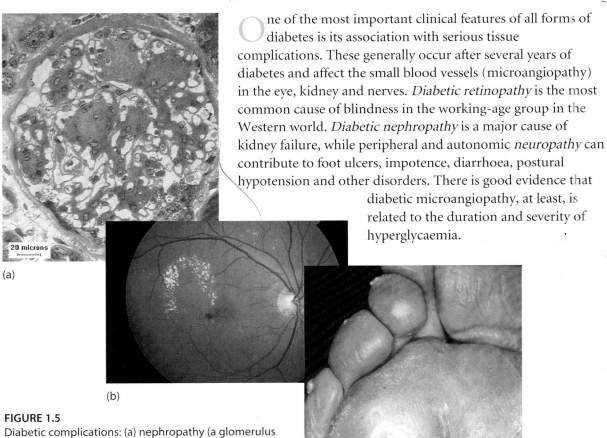

20 microns

(a)

(b)

(c)

FIGURE 1.5
Diabetic complications: (a) nephropathy (a glomerulus showing nodular sclerosis), (b) diabetic retinopathy and (c) a typical neuropathic foot ulcer.

The frequency of arterial disease (atherosclerosis or macroangiopathy) is also markedly increased in diabetic people and is responsible for an excess of coronary heart disease, strokes and peripheral vascular disease – the lower-limb amputation rate is over 15-fold higher in the diabetic than in the general population.

Diabetes is a common disease, with major global health consequences. There are particularly high frequencies in ethnic minorities living in industrial or Westernized societies, such as Native Americans in the USA and Indian Asians in the UK. We are witnessing a worldwide epidemic of diabetes; the current prevalence is at least 150 million people, a figure that is predicted to double by the year 2025. In the future, most cases will be in developing countries that are adopting a Westernized lifestyle.

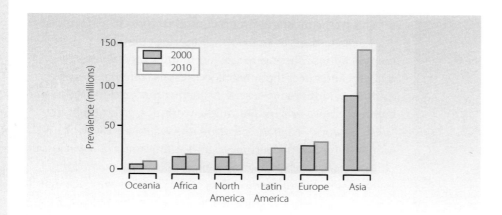

FIGURE 1.6
Estimated prevalence of diabetes in various regions of the world, in 2000 and predicted for 2010.

HISTORY OF DIABETES

2

Diseases with the clinical features of diabetes have been recognized since antiquity. The Ebers papyrus, dating from 1550 BC, describes a polyuric state that resembles diabetes. (The papyrus was discovered in 1862 by the German Egyptologist, Georg Ebers).

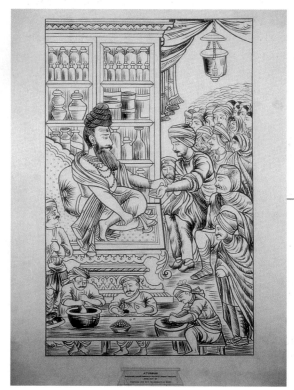

FIGURE 2.1
The Ebers papyrus.

The word 'diabetes' was first used by Aretaeus of Cappadocia in the 2nd century AD. It comes from the Greek, meaning *siphon* ('because the fluid does not remain in the body, but uses the man's body as a channel whereby to leave it'). Aretaeus gave a clinical description of the disease, noting the increased urine flow, thirst and weight loss, features that are instantly recognizable today.

Diabetes is a dreadful affliction, not very frequent among men, being a melting down of the flesh and limbs into urine. The patients never stop making water and the flow is incessant, like the opening of aqueducts. Life is short, unpleasant and painful, thirst unquenchable, drinking excessive, and disproportionate to the large quantity of urine, for yet more urine is passed. One cannot stop them either from drinking or making water. If for a while they abstain from drinking, their mouths become parched and their bodies dry; the viscera seem scorched up, the patients are affected by nausea, restlessness and a burning thirst, and within a short time, they expire.

FIGURE 2.2
Description of diabetes by Aretaeus.

The sweet, honey-like taste of urine in polyuric states, which attracted ants and other insects, was reported by Hindu physicians such as Sushrut (Susruta) during the 5th and 6th century AD. These descriptions even mention two forms of diabetes, the more common occurring in older, overweight and indolent people, and the other in lean people who did not survive for long. This empirical subdivision predicted the modern classification into type 1 and type 2 diabetes.

FIGURE 2.3
Susruta, an Indian physician.

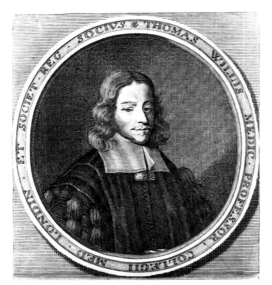

FIGURE 2.4
Thomas Willis.

Diabetes was largely neglected in Europe until the 17th century English physician, Thomas Willis (1621–1675), rediscovered the sweetness of diabetic urine. Willis, who was physician to King Charles II, thought that the disease had been rare in ancient times, but that its frequency was increasing in his age 'given to good fellowship'. Nearly a century later, the Liverpool physician, Matthew Dobson (1735–1784) showed that the sweetness of urine and serum was caused by sugar. John Rollo (d. 1809) was the first to apply the adjective 'mellitus' to the disease (Greek and Latin for 'honey').

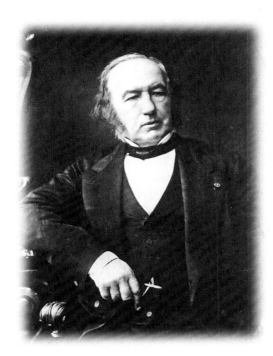

FIGURE 2.5
Claude Bernard.

In the 19th century, the French physiologist, Claude Bernard (1813–1878) made many discoveries relating to diabetes. Among these was the finding that the sugar that appears in the urine was stored in the liver as glycogen.

Bernard also demonstrated links between the central nervous system and diabetes when he observed temporary hyperglycaemia (*piqûre* diabetes) when the medulla of conscious rabbits was transfixed with a needle.

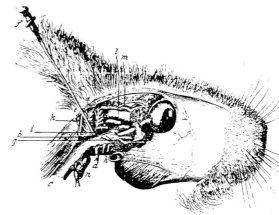

FIGURE 2.6
Piqûre diabetes.

In 1889, Oskar Minkowski (1858–1931) and Joseph von Mering (1849-1908) from Strasbourg removed the pancreas from a dog to see if the organ was essential for life. The animal displayed typical signs of diabetes, with thirst, polyuria and wasting, which were associated with glycosuria and hyperglycaemia. This experiment showed that a pancreatic disorder causes diabetes, but they did not follow up on the observation.

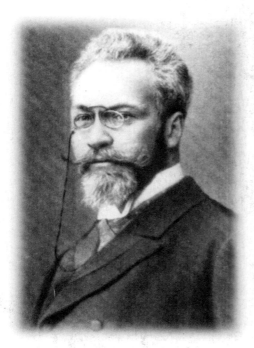

FIGURE 2.7
Oskar Minkowski.

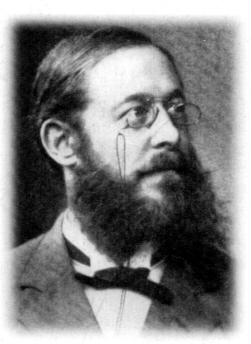

FIGURE 2.8
Josef von Mering.

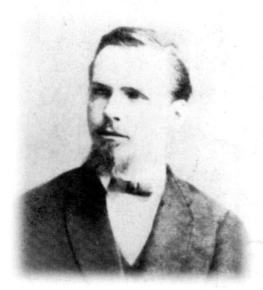

FIGURE 2.9
Paul Langerhans.

Paul Langerhans (1847–1888) from Berlin was the first to describe (in his doctoral thesis of 1869) small clusters of cells in teased preparations of the pancreas. He did not speculate on the function of the cells, and it was Edouard Laguesse in France who later (1893) named the cells 'islets of Langerhans' and suggested that they were endocrine tissue of the pancreas that produced a glucose-lowering hormone.

HANDBOOK OF DIABETES 3RD EDITION

In the early 20th century, several workers isolated impure hypoglycaemic extracts from the pancreas, including the Berlin physician Georg Zuelzer (1840–1949), the Romanian Nicolas Paulesco (1869–1931), and the Americans Ernest Scott (1877–1966) and Israel Kleiner.

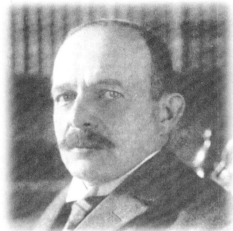

FIGURE 2.10
Georg Zuelzer.

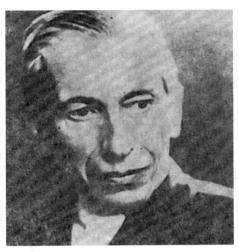

FIGURE 2.11
Nicolas Paulesco.

Insulin was discovered in 1921 at the University of Toronto, Canada, through a collaboration between the surgeon Frederick G Banting (1891–1941), his student assistant Charles H Best (1899–1978), the biochemist James B Collip (1892–1965) and the physiologist JJR Macleod (1876–1935).

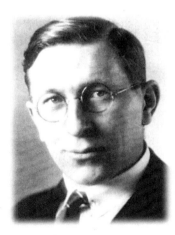

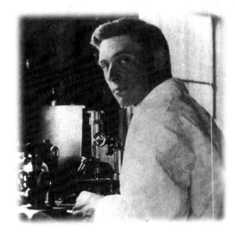

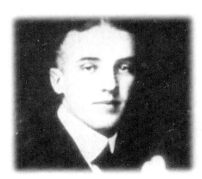

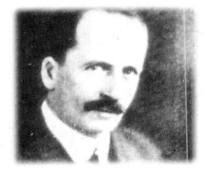

FIGURE 2.12
The discoverers of insulin. Clockwise from top left: Frederick G. Banting, James B. Collip, J.J.R. Macleod and Charles H. Best.

Banting and Best made chilled extracts of dog pancreas, injected them into pancreactectomized diabetic dogs, and showed a decline in blood sugar concentrations.

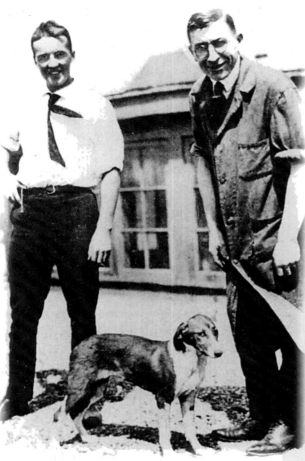

FIGURE 2.13
Charles Best and Frederick Banting in Toronto in 1922 (the dog is thought to have been called Marjorie).

Banting and Best's notes of the dog experiments refer to the administration of 'isletin', later called insulin by them at the suggestion of Macleod. They were unaware that the Belgian Jean de Meyer had already coined the term 'insuline' in 1909. (All these names ultimately derive from the Latin for 'island').

FIGURE 2.14
Banting and Best's notebook.

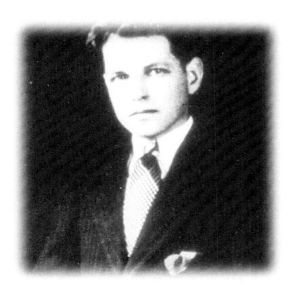

FIGURE 2.15
Leonard Thompson.

Collip improved the methods for the extraction and purification of insulin from the pancreas, and the first diabetic patient, a 14-year-old boy called Leonard Thompson, was treated on 11th January 1922. A commercially viable extraction procedure was then developed in collaboration with chemists from Eli Lilly and Co. in the USA, and insulin became widely available in North America and Europe from 1923. The 1923 Nobel Prize for Physiology or Medicine was awarded to Banting and Macleod, who decided to share their prizes with Best and Collip.

The American physician Elliot P Joslin (1869–1962) was one of the first doctors to gain experience with insulin. Working in Boston, he treated 293 patients in the first year after August 1922. Joslin also introduced systematic education for his diabetic patients and became arguably the most famous diabetes specialist of the 20th century.

In the UK, the discovery of insulin saved the life of the London physician Robin D Lawrence (1892–1968), who had recently developed type 1 diabetes. He subsequently played a leading part in the founding of the British Diabetic Association (now Diabetes UK).

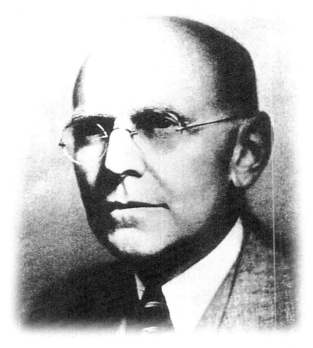

FIGURE 2.16
Elliot P. Joslin.

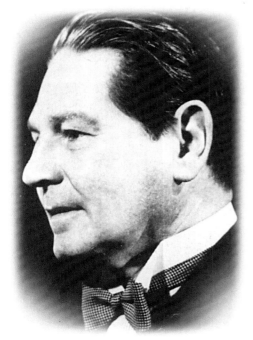

FIGURE 2.17
Robin D. Lawrence.

11

HANDBOOK OF DIABETES 3RD EDITION

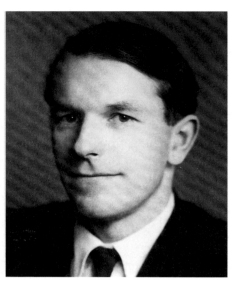

FIGURE 2.18
Frederick Sanger.

Among the many major advances since the introduction of insulin into clinical practice was the elucidation in 1955 of its primary structure (amino acid sequence) by the Cambridge UK scientist, Frederick Sanger (b. 1918), who received the Nobel Prize for this work in 1958.

Oxford-based Dorothy Hodgkin (1910–1994), another Nobel Prize winner, and her colleagues described the three-dimensional structure of insulin using X-ray crystallography (1969).

By the 1950s, it was accepted that tissue complications, such as occur in the eye and kidney, continued to develop in long-standing diabetes, in spite of insulin treatment. The definitive proof that normalization of glycaemia could prevent or delay the development of diabetic complications had to wait until 1993 for type 1 diabetes [the Diabetes Control and Complications Trial (DCCT) in North America] and 1998 for type 2 diabetes (the UK Prospective Diabetes Study, UKPDS). The UKPDS was initiated and directed by the Oxford physician, Robert Turner (1939–1999).

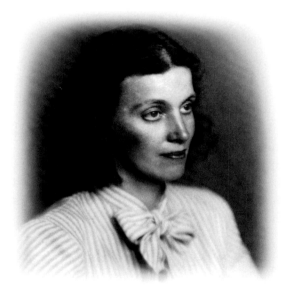

FIGURE 2.19
Dorothy Hodgkin.

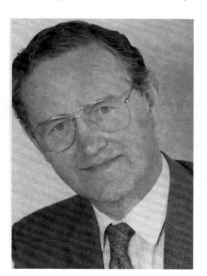

FIGURE 2.20
Robert Turner, instigator of the UKPDS, which proved that good control of blood glucose and blood pressure was beneficial in type 2 diabetes.

DIAGNOSIS AND CLASSIFICATION OF DIABETES

3

Diabetes mellitus is diagnosed by identifying chronic hyperglycaemia. The diagnostic criteria and classification proposed during the 1970s by the World Health Organization (WHO) were widely accepted until 1997, when the American Diabetes Association (ADA) suggested new criteria; these were essentially ratified by the WHO in 1999. The diagnostic thresholds are defined from epidemiological studies of the natural history of glucose intolerance, particularly the concentrations of blood glucose associated with diabetes-specific microvascular complications, such as retinopathy and nephropathy.

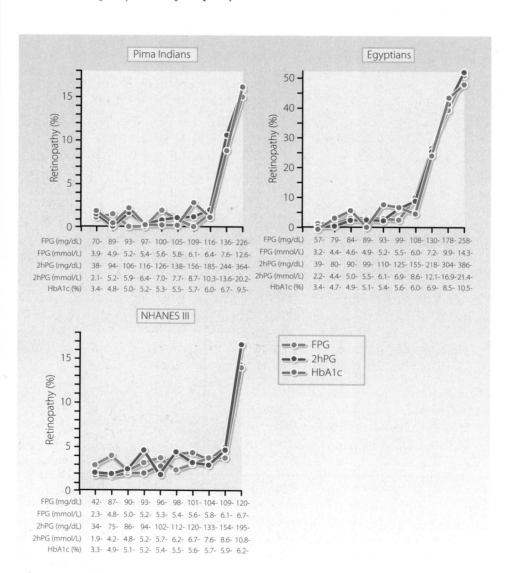

FIGURE 3.1
Prevalence of retinopathy in 3 populations: the Pima Indians in the USA (who have a high frequency of diabetes), Egyptians and participants in the NHANES III study in the USA. Note that in each case retinopathy is associated with a fasting plasma glucose (FPG) level greater than about 7 mmol/L (126 mg/dL) and a plasma glucose 2 hours after an oral glucose load (2hPG) of greater than about 11 mmol/L (200 mg/dL). Glycated haemoglobin (HbA$_{1c}$) concentrations show similar relationships.

In the latest ADA–WHO diagnostic criteria, diabetes can be diagnosed in three ways:

- In subjects with clinical symptoms and signs of diabetes, by a casual (random) plasma glucose ≥ 11.1 mmol/L (200 mg/dL).
- By a fasting plasma glucose ≥ 7.0 mmol/L (126 mg/dL).
- By a plasma glucose ≥ 11.1 mmol/L (200 mg/dL), 2 hours after a 75 g load of glucose given by mouth [the oral glucose tolerance test (OGTT)].

The hyperglycaemia should be confirmed on a subsequent day by any of the three methods. The WHO recommends that the OGTT be used for diagnosis when the random plasma glucose is in the uncertain range, between 5.5 and 11.1 mmol/L (100–200 mg/dL).

ADA Diagnostic criteria, 1997

1 Symptoms + random plasma glucose ≥11.1 mmol/L (≥200 mg/dL)

2 Fasting plasma glucose ≥7.0 mmol/L (≥126 mg/dL)

3 75g OGTT 2 h plasma glucose ≥11.1 mmol/L (≥200 mg/dL)

- Each method confirmed on a subsequent day by any method

- Impaired fasting glucose (IFG) ≥6.1 and <7.0 mmol/L (≥110 and <126 mg/dL)

FIGURE 3.2
Diagnostic criteria for diabetes. (To convert glucose concentrations in mmol/L into mg/dL, multiply by 18.)

Intermediate categories of hyperglycaemia

During the natural history of all forms of diabetes, the disease passes through a stage of *impaired glucose tolerance* (IGT), defined as a plasma glucose ≥ 7.8 and < 11.1 mmol/L (140–200 mg/dL) 2 hours after an OGTT.

Impaired fasting glucose (IFG) is an analogous category based on fasting glucose levels, and is defined as a fasting plasma glucose ≥ 6.1 mmol/L and < 7.0 mmol/L (110–126 mg/dL).

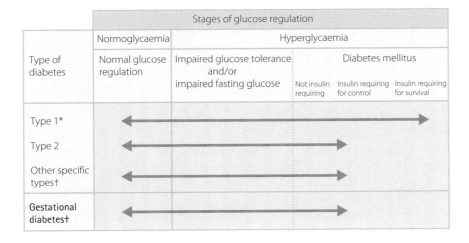

FIGURE 3.3
The stages of glucose regulation in different types of diabetes. Impaired glucose tolerance and/or impaired fasting glucose is a stage through which patients pass before developing diabetes. *Type 1 diabetic patients can briefly return to normoglycaemia shortly after diagnosis – the 'honeymoon period'. †In rare cases (e.g. type 1 diabetes presenting in pregnancy), patients may require insulin for survival.

IGT and/or IFG

- A stage in the natural history of disordered glucose metabolism
- Can lead to any type of diabetes
- Increased risk of progression to diabetes
- Increased risk of cardiovascular disease
- Little or no risk of microvascular disease
- Some patients may revert to normoglycaemia

FIGURE 3.4
Some features of impaired glucose tolerance and/or impaired fasting glucose.

IGT and IFG are sometimes regarded as forms of 'borderline diabetes'. Unlike diabetes, these categories of glucose intolerance are not associated with microvascular disease, but do carry increased risk of cardiovascular disease. IGT is not a permanent state: some subjects with IGT progress to diabetes, while others may revert to normoglycaemia.

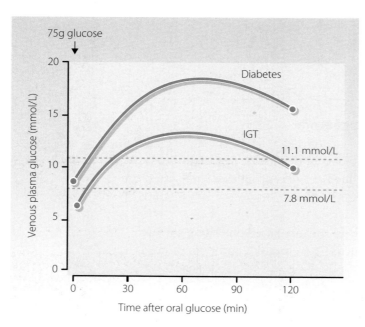

FIGURE 3.5
Diagnosis of diabetes and IGT by the oral glucose tolerance test.

For the OGTT, the subject is tested in the morning after an overnight fast, in the seated position and having refrained from smoking. After taking a fasting blood sample, 75 g of glucose is given by mouth, often in the form of a glucose drink such as Lucozade (388 mL). For children, the glucose dose is calculated as 1.75 g/kg. A further blood sample is taken at 2 hours, and the fasting and 2-hour glucose values are interpreted as in *Figure 3.5*.

HANDBOOK OF DIABETES 3RD EDITION

Glycosuria (the presence of glucose in the urine) is responsible for the classic diabetic symptoms and was previously regarded as a diagnostic hallmark of the disease. Nowadays, it indicates the need to test blood glucose, but cannot be used to diagnose diabetes because of the poor relationship between blood and urine glucose (*Figure 3.6*). This is for several reasons: the renal threshold for glucose reabsorption varies considerably within and between individuals, the urine glucose concentration is affected by the subject's state of hydration and the result reflects the average blood glucose during the period that urine has accumulated in the bladder. The average *renal threshold* is 10 mmol/L (i.e. a blood glucose concentration above this level 'spills over' into the urine), but a negative urine test can be associated with marked hyperglycaemia.

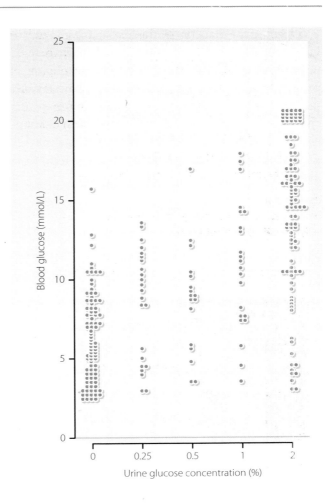

FIGURE 3.6
Simultaneous blood and urinary glucose concentrations obtained from diabetic children.

Longer term indices of hyperglycaemia include the glycated haemoglobin percentage (HbA$_{1c}$), a measure of integrated blood glucose control over the preceding few weeks (see Chapter 9). This is used primarily to assess glycaemic control and adjust treatment in diabetic patients; it may provide useful confirmatory information for the screening and diagnosis of diabetes, but cannot be used on its own for the diagnosis of the disease.

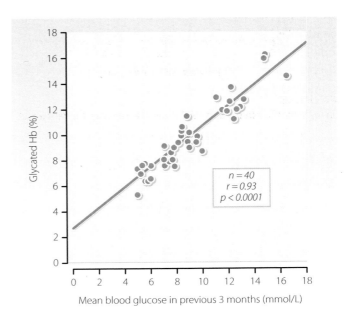

FIGURE 3.7
HbA$_{1c}$ correlates well with previous mean blood glucose levels but is not used to diagnose diabetes.

Screening for diabetes by the fasting plasma glucose does not identify exactly the same population as that diagnosed by the plasma glucose 2 hours after an OGTT (*Figure 3.8*). The overlap depends on the ethnic and geographical population, and on other characteristics such as age. Some individuals have asymptomatic, isolated post-challenge hyperglycaemia, while others have fasting hyperglycaemia but normal post-load glycaemic responses. The fasting criteria for diabetes tend to pick out younger and more obese subjects.

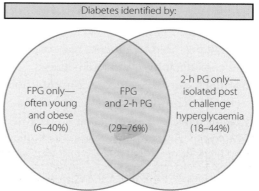

FIGURE 3.8
Screening for diabetes by fasting plasma glucose (FPG ≥ 7.0 mmol/L) or by plasma glucose (2 h PG ≥ 11.1 mmol/L) after an oral glucose tolerance test identifies different populations of subjects.

The potential value of screening for diabetes is early diagnosis and treatment. About 20% of newly diagnosed type 2 diabetic subjects already have tissue complications, such as retinopathy, the prevalence of which increases with diabetes duration. This suggests that complications begin about 5–6 years before diagnosis and the actual onset of diabetes may be 10 years or more before usual clinical diagnosis.

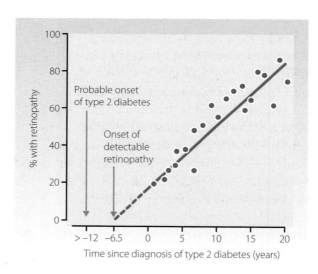

FIGURE 3.9
The prevalence of retinopathy in type 2 diabetes relative to the time of clinical diagnosis. Note the presence of retinopathy at diagnosis and the likely onset of retinopathy and diabetes some years before diagnosis.

HANDBOOK OF DIABETES 3RD EDITION

Population studies have also shown that many people have undiagnosed type 2 diabetes and IGT. Within any age group, there are probably approximately equal numbers of diagnosed and undiagnosed people with diabetes. 'Preclinical' type 2 diabetes is associated with many modifiable risk factors for ill health, in addition to hyperglycaemia, such as obesity, hyperlipidaemia, hypertension and cigarette smoking.

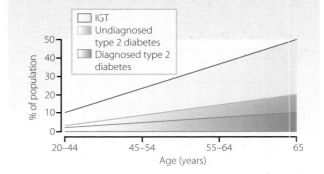

FIGURE 3.10
Estimated prevalence of diagnosed and undiagnosed diabetes and impaired glucose tolerance (IGT) in the USA. Note that for any age group, there are about equal numbers of diagnosed and undiagnosed people with diabetes.

In most countries, screening methods have not yet been agreed. The fasting plasma glucose is simple, quick, acceptable to patients and of low cost, but can miss those with isolated post-challenge hyperglycaemia. The OGTT is more difficult to perform, impractical for large numbers and expensive, but is the only way to identify post-load hyperglycaemia. Methods, benefits and risks of screening are all being evaluated. At present, attention is focused on those at high risk of developing diabetes.

High-risk categories

The obese, especially those with truncal obesity

Those with parents or siblings with type 2 diabetes

Those over 45 years of age

Ethnic minorities with increased risk

Those with existing coronary heart, cerebrovascular, or peripheral vascular disease, or hypertension

Those with dyslipidaemia

Women with a history of gestational diabetes or delivery of large babies

Women with polycystic ovary disease who are obese

Those with known IGT/IFG

FIGURE 3.11
Some 'high-risk' individuals who would be appropriate for targeted screening programmes. Two or more risk factors may be required.

Classification of diabetes
Type 1 (β-cell destruction, usually leading to absolute insulin deficiency)
• Autoimmune
• Idiopathic
Type 2
• Ranges from predominantly insulin-resistant, with relative insulin deficiency, to a predominantly insulin-secretory defect, with or without insulin resistance
Other specific types
• Genetic defects of β-cell function
• Genetic defects of insulin action
• Diseases of exocrine pancreas
• Endocrinopathies
• Drug-induced or chemical-induced
• Infections
• Uncommon forms of immune-mediated diabetes
• Other genetic syndromes sometimes associated with diabetes
Gestational diabetes

FIGURE 3.12
Classification of diabetes.

IDDM	NIDDM
Type 1	Type 2
LADA (late stage)	LADA (early stage)

FIGURE 3.13
Type 1 and 2 diabetes are equivalent to IDDM and NIDDM.

The current classification of diabetes is based on the aetiology of the disease. There are four categories:

- *Type 1 diabetes* (caused by pancreatic islet cell destruction).
- *Type 2 diabetes* (caused insulin resistance and a β-cell insulin secretory defect, which occur in varying proportions).
- *Other specific types of diabetes* [caused by such conditions such as endocrinopathies, diseases of the exocrine pancreas, genetic syndromes, etc. (see below)].
- *Gestational diabetes* (defined as diabetes that occurs for the first time in pregnancy).

Type 1 diabetes is subdivided into two main types: *1a* or *autoimmune* (about 90% of type 1 patients in Europe and North America, in which immune markers, such as circulating islet cell antibodies, suggest autoimmune destruction of the β cells); and *1b* or *idiopathic* (where there is no evidence of autoimmunity).

This classification has now replaced the earlier, clinical classification into 'insulin-dependent diabetes mellitus' (IDDM) and 'non-insulin-dependent diabetes mellitus' (NIDDM), which was based on the need for insulin treatment at diagnosis. IDDM is broadly equivalent to type 1 diabetes and NIDDM to type 2 diabetes. One of the disadvantages of the classification according to treatment was that subjects could change their type of diabetes – for example, some type 1a patients diagnosed after the age of 40 years appear to have NIDDM, before eventually becoming truly insulin-dependent (this is now classified as *latent autoimmune diabetes in adults*, LADA).

Type 1 diabetes	Type 2 diabetes
Sudden onset	Gradual onset
Severe symptoms, including ketoacidotic coma in some	May be no symptoms
Recent weight loss	Often no weight loss
Usually lean	Usually obese
Spontaneous ketosis	Not ketotic
Absent C peptide	C peptide detectable
Markers of autoimmunity present (e.g. islet cell antibodies)	No markers of autoimmunity

Various clinical and biochemical features can be used to decide whether the patient has type 1 or type 2 diabetes. The distinction may be difficult in individual cases.

FIGURE 3.14
Type 1 or type 2 diabetes?

The category of 'other specific types of diabetes' is a large group of conditions, which includes genetic defects in insulin secretion [such as in maturity-onset diabetes of the young (MODY) and insulinopathies], genetic defects in insulin action (e.g. syndromes of severe insulin resistance), pancreatitis and other exocrine disorders, hormone-secreting tumours such as acromegaly (growth hormone) and Cushing's syndrome (cortisol). Some cases are caused by the administration of drugs, notably glucocorticoids. Some genetic syndromes are sometimes associated with diabetes (e.g. Down's syndrome, Klinefelter's syndrome and many more).

Genetic defects of β-cell function
Chromosome 12, HNF-1α (formerly MODY-3)
Chromosome 7, glucokinase (formerly MODY-2)
Chromosome 20, HNF-4α (formerly MODY-1)
Mitochondrial DNA
Insulinopathies

Genetic defects in insulin action
Type A insulin resistance
Leprechaunism
Rabson–Mendenhall syndrome
Lipoatrophic diabetes

Diseases of the exocrine pancreas
Pancreatitis
Trauma/pancreatectomy
Neoplasia
Cystic fibrosis
Haemochromatosis
Fibrocalculous pancreatopathy

Endocrinopathies
Acromegaly
Cushing's syndrome
Glucagonoma
Phaeochromocytoma
Hyperthyroidism
Somatostatinoma
Aldosteronoma

Drug-induced or chemical-induced
Glucocorticoids
Thiazides
Vacor
Pentamidine
Nicotinic acid
Glucocorticoids
Thyroid hormone
Diazoxide
β-adrenergic agonists
Dilantin
Interferon-α

Infections
Congenital rubella
Cytomegalovirus
Others
Uncommon forms of immune-mediated diabetes
'Stiff man' syndrome
Anti-insulin receptor antibodies

Other genetic syndromes sometimes associated with diabetes
Down's syndrome
Klinefelter's syndrome
Turner's syndrome
Wolfram's syndrome
Friedreich's ataxia
Huntington's chorea
Lawrence–Moon–Biedl syndrome
Myotonic dystrophy
Porphyria
Prader–Willi syndrome

FIGURE 3.15
Other specific types of diabetes.

PUBLIC HEALTH ASPECTS OF DIABETES 4

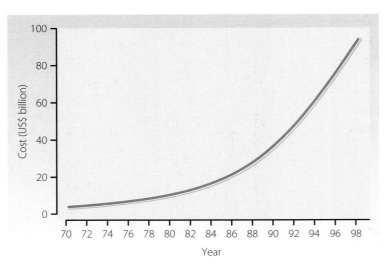

FIGURE 4.1
The rising costs of diabetes in the USA.

Diabetes is an expensive disease, accounting for at least 5% of the total health-care costs in European countries. About 75% of the direct costs are absorbed by the long-term complications, rather than the management of diabetes itself. In the USA, the direct costs (treatment, diagnosis, care etc) and indirect costs (lost output due to disability, premature death etc) were each about US$50 billion in the late 1990s. About 90% of resources for diabetes care are spent on type 2 diabetes. Even accounting for inflation, the cost of diabetes is increasing year on year.

	Type 1 (%)	Type 2 (%)
Cardiovascular disease	15	58
Cerebrovascular disease	3	12
Nephropathy	55	3
Diabetic coma	4	1
Malignancy	0	11
Infections	10	4
Others	13	11

The overall life expectancy in the diabetic person is reduced by about 25%. The causes of death differ between type 1 and type 2 diabetes. In long-duration type 1 diabetes, nephropathy and heart disease are common, whereas in type 2 diabetes most deaths are due to cardiovascular disease.

FIGURE 4.2
Causes of mortality in type 1 and type 2 diabetes.

In recent years, mortality rates from type 1 diabetes have been falling in many countries, probably because of better blood glucose and blood pressure control.

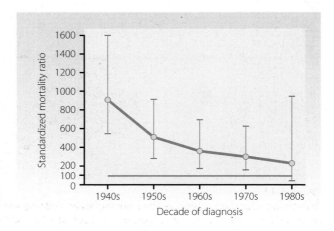

FIGURE 4.3
Falling mortality in type 1 diabetes. From a cohort of 845 people diagnosed with diabetes before the age of 17 years in Leicestershire, UK, between 1940 and 1989. Vertical bars are 95% confidence intervals. 100 = national mortality rate.

Diabetes is a serious global health problem, and one that is going to become much worse. It already affects at least 5-7% of the world's population, and its prevalence is expected to increase from about 135 million people in 1995 to 300 million people by 2025; 90% of these people will have type 2 diabetes.

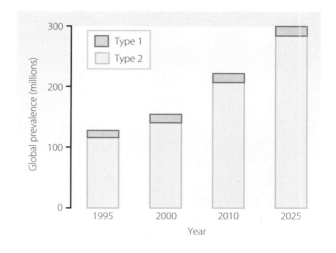

FIGURE 4.4
Estimated worldwide prevalences of type 1 and type 2 diabetes, 1995–2025

The frequency of diabetes is rising, especially in developing countries, where the lifestyle has changed from one based on traditional, agricultural subsistence to a westernized, urban culture. Readily available high-energy foods and physical inactivity lead to obesity and to diabetes in these susceptible populations. Many diabetic patients in developing countries present late with serious infections or tissue complications. Diabetic emergencies have a high mortality. Practical difficulties in developing countries include lack of doctors, nurses and dietitians and shortages of drugs, including insulin.

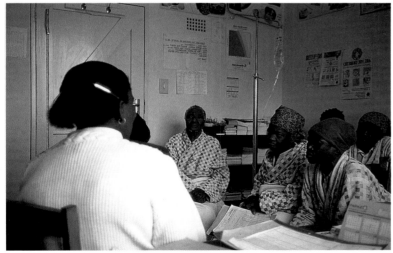

FIGURE 4.5
A morning education session, led by a nursing sister, at Baragwanath Hospital in Soweto, South Africa. All these patients had been admitted with diabetic emergencies during the preceding 24 hours.

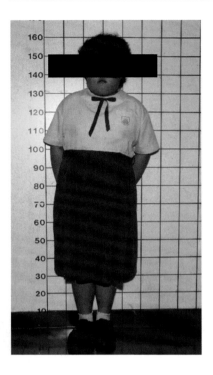

Traditionally, type 2 diabetes has been a disease of the middle-aged and the elderly, but it is now becoming a problem among adolescents and even children. A sedentary lifestyle and obesity are the main contributory factors, though many have a positive family history of type 2 diabetes. In some parts of the USA, type 2 diabetes now accounts for one-third of new cases of diabetes in adolescence, while 80% of diabetic children and adolescents in Japan suffer from type 2 diabetes.

FIGURE 4.6
An 11-year-old girl from Hong Kong with type 2 diabetes. Note the marked truncal obesity.

The global type 2 diabetes epidemic, which is driven mainly by obesity and physical inactivity, is potentially preventable by the institution of appropriate public health measures in communities or in high-risk groups. Recent studies have shown that lifestyle measures can prevent the progression of IGT to overt type 2 diabetes. In the Finnish Diabetes Prevention Study, for example, an individualized programme that comprises a weight-reducing, high-fibre, low-fat diet with increased physical exercise reduced by 58% the risk of overweight subjects with IGT progressing to diabetes.

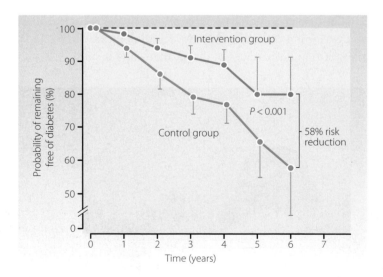

FIGURE 4.7
Diet and exercise (intervention group), reduces the progression of IGT to type 2 diabetes (Finnish Diabetes Prevention Study).

NORMAL PHYSIOLOGY OF INSULIN SECRETION AND ACTION

5

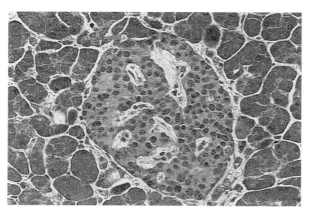

FIGURE 5.1

A section of normal pancreas stained with haematoxylin and eosin. The islet in the centre is identified easily by its distinct morphology and lighter staining than that of the surrounding exocrine tissue (original magnification ×350).

Insulin is synthesized in and secreted from the β cells within the islets of Langerhans in the pancreas. The normal pancreas has about 1 million islets, which constitute about 2–3% of the gland's mass. All of the islet cell-types are derived embryologically from endodermal outgrowths of the fetal gut. The islets can be identified easily with various histological stains, such as haematoxylin and eosin, with which the cells react less intensely than does the surrounding exocrine tissue. The islets vary in size from a few dozen to several thousands of cells and are scattered irregularly throughout the exocrine pancreas.

The main cell types of the pancreas are β cells (producing insulin), α cells (producing glucagon), δ cells (producing somatostatin) and PP cells (producing pancreatic polypeptide). The different cell types can be identified in various ways, including immunostaining techniques, *in-situ* hybridization for their hormone products (using nucleotide probes complementary to the target mRNA) and the electron-microscope appearance of their secretory granules. The β cells are the most numerous type and are located mainly in the core of the islet, while α and δ cells are located in the periphery.

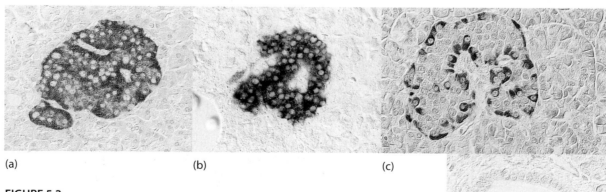

(a)   (b)   (c)

FIGURE 5.2

The localization of pancreatic hormones in human islets. (a) Insulin immunostained in the majority of cells that form the core of the islet (peroxidase–antiperoxidase immunostain with haematoxylin counterstain). (b) Insulin mRNA localized by *in situ* hybridization with a digoxigenin-labelled sequence of rat insulin cRNA (which cross-reacts fully with human insulin mRNA). (c) Peripherally located α cells immunostained with antibodies to pancreatic glucagon using the same method as for (a). (d) Weakly immunoreactive PP cells in the epithelium of a duct in the ventral portion of the pancreatic head. Magnifications approximately ×150.

(d)

Islets cells interact with each other through direct contact and through their products (e.g. glucagon stimulates insulin secretion, while somatostatin inhibits insulin and glucagon secretion). The blood flow within the islets is organized centrifugally so that the different cell types are supplied in the sequence β→α→δ. Insulin also has an 'autocrine' (self-regulating) effect that alters the transcription of insulin and glucokinase genes in the β cell.

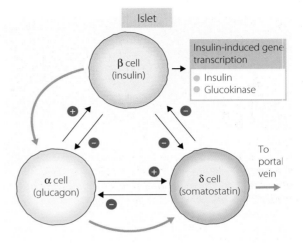

FIGURE 5.3
Potential interactions between the secretory products of the major islet-cell types. Black arrows indicate paracrine stimulation or inhibition. The direction of blood flow within the islet is indicated by the red arrows.

The islets are densely innervated with autonomic and peptidergic nerves. Parasympathetic innervation from the vagus stimulates insulin release, while adrenergic sympathetic nerves inhibit insulin and stimulate glucagon secretion. Other nerves that originate within the pancreas contain peptides such as vasoactive intestinal peptide (VIP), which stimulates the release of all islet hormones, and neuropeptide Y (NPY), which inhibits insulin secretion. The overall importance of these neuropeptides in controlling islet-cell secretion remains unclear.

FIGURE 5.4
Structure of a pancreatic islet, showing the anatomical relationships between the four major endocrine cell types. NPY, neuropeptide Y; VIP, vasoactive intestinal polypeptide.

The insulin molecule consists of two polypeptide chains, linked by disulphide bridges; the A chain contains 21 amino acids and the B chain 30 amino acids. Human insulin differs from pig insulin, an animal insulin which has been used extensively for diabetes treatment, at only one amino acid position (B30). Beef insulin (also used therapeutically) differs at three positions (B30, A8 and A10).

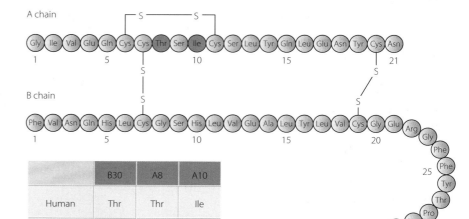

FIGURE 5.5
The primary structure (amino-acid sequence) of human insulin. The highlighted residues are those that differ in porcine and bovine insulins, as shown in the inset.

	B30	A8	A10
Human	Thr	Thr	Ile
Porcine	Ala	Thr	Ile
Bovine	Ala	Ala	Val

In dilute solution and in the circulation, insulin exists as a monomer of 6000 Da molecular weight. The tertiary (three-dimensional) structure of monomeric insulin consists of a hydrophobic core buried beneath a surface that is hydrophilic, except for two non-polar regions involved in the aggregation of the monomers into dimers and hexamers. In concentrated solution (such as in the insulin vial supplied by the pharmaceutical company for injection) and in crystals (such as in the insulin secretory granule), six monomers self-associate with two zinc ions to form a hexamer. This is of therapeutic importance because the slow absorption of native insulin from the subcutaneous tissue partly results from the time taken for the hexameric insulin to dissociate into the smaller, more easily absorbed monomeric form (see Chapter 10).

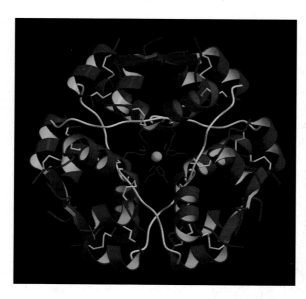

FIGURE 5.6
The double zinc insulin hexamer composed of three insulin dimers in a threefold symmetrical pattern.

Insulin is synthesized in the islet β cells from a single amino acid chain precursor molecule called proinsulin. Synthesis begins with the formation of an even larger precursor, preproinsulin, which is cleaved by protease activity to proinsulin. The gene for preproinsulin (and therefore the 'gene for insulin') is located on chromosome 11. Proinsulin is packaged into vesicles in the Golgi apparatus of the β cell; in the maturing secretory granules that bud off it, proinsulin is converted by enzymes into insulin and connecting peptide (C peptide).

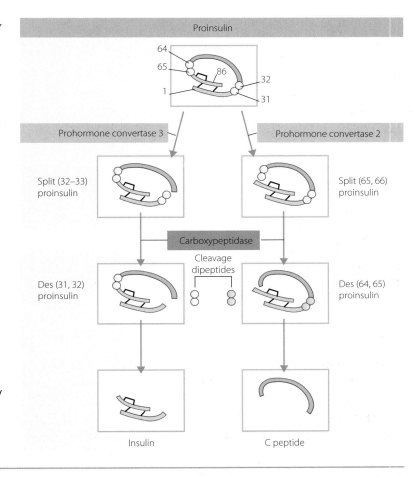

FIGURE 5.7
Insulin biosynthesis and processing. Proinsulin is cleaved on the C-terminal side of two dipeptides. The cleavage dipeptides are liberated, so yielding the 'split' proinsulin products and ultimately insulin and C peptide.

Insulin and C peptide are released from the β cell when the granules are transported ('translocated') to the cell surface and fuse with the plasma membrane (exocytosis). Microtubules, formed of polymerized tubulin, probably provide the mechanical framework for granule transport and microfilaments of actin, interacting with myosin and other motor proteins such as kinesin, may provide the motive force that propels the granules along the tubules.

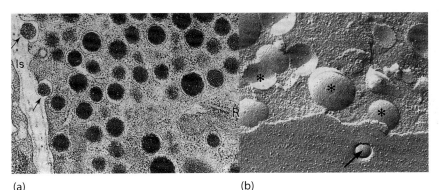

(a) (b)

FIGURE 5.8
(a) Electron micrograph of insulin secretory granules in a pancreatic β cell and their secretion by exocytosis. Arrows show exocytosis occurring. Ca, capillary lumen; Is, interstitial space. (b) Freeze-fracture views of β cells that reveal the secretory granules in the cytoplasm (asterisks) and the granule content released by exocytosis at the cell membrane (arrows). Magnification: ×52 000.

This 'regulated pathway', with almost complete cleavage of proinsulin to insulin, normally carries about 95% of the β cell insulin production. In certain conditions, such as insulinoma and type 2 diabetes, an alternative 'constitutive' pathway operates, in which large amounts of unprocessed proinsulin and intermediate insulin precursors ('split proinsulins') are released directly from vesicles that originate in the endoplasmic reticulum.

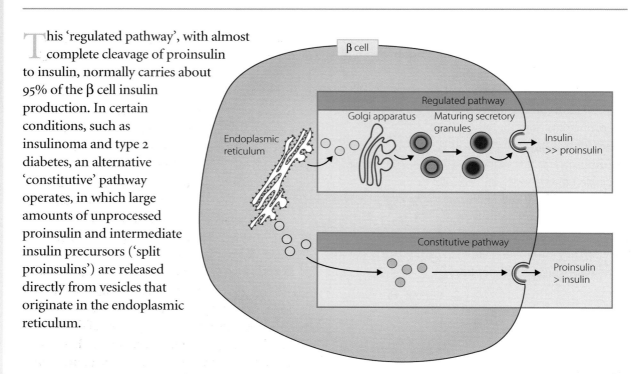

FIGURE 5.9
The regulated (normal) and constitutive (active in type 2 diabetes) pathways of insulin processing.

Glucose is the main stimulator of insulin release from the β cell, which occurs in a characteristic biphasic pattern – an acute first phase that lasts only a few minutes, followed by a sustained second phase. The shape of the glucose–insulin dose–response curve is determined primarily by the activity of glucokinase, which governs the rate-limiting step for glucose metabolism in the β cell (see below). Glucose levels below about 4 mmol/L (72 mg/dL) do not induce insulin release; half-maximal stimulation occurs at about 8 mmol/L (144 mg/dL).

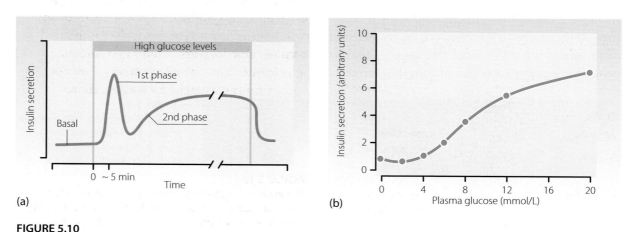

FIGURE 5.10
(a) The biphasic glucose-stimulated release of insulin from the islets. (b) The glucose–insulin dose–response curve for islets of Langerhans.

HANDBOOK OF DIABETES 3RD EDITION

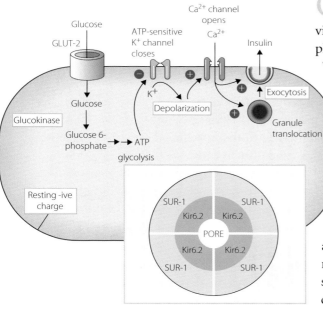

FIGURE 5.11

The mechanism of glucose-stimulated insulin secretion from the β cell. The structure of the K$_{ATP}$ channel is shown in the inset.

Glucose must be metabolized within the β cell to stimulate insulin secretion. It enters the β cell via the GLUT-2 transporter (see below) and is then phosphorylated by glucokinase, which acts as the 'glucose sensor' that couples insulin secretion to the prevailing glucose level. Glycolysis and mitochondrial metabolism produce adenosine triphosphatase (ATP), which closes ATP-sensitive potassium (K$_{ATP}$) channels. This causes depolarization of the β-cell plasma membrane, which leads to an influx of extracellular calcium through voltage-gated channels in the membrane. The increase in cytosolic calcium triggers granule translocation and exocytosis. Sulphonylureas (drugs used in the management of type 2 diabetes) stimulate insulin secretion by binding to a component of the K$_{ATP}$ channel (the sulphonylurea receptor, SUR-1) and closing it (see Chapter 11). The K$_{ATP}$ channel is an octamer that consists of four K$^+$-channel subunits (called Kir6.2) and four SUR-1 subunits.

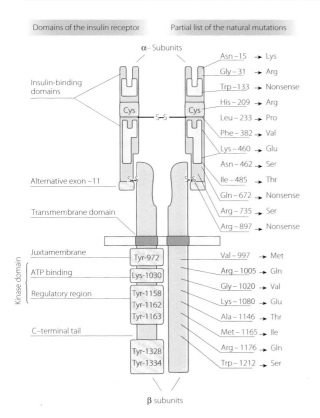

Insulin exerts its main biological effects by binding to a cell-surface receptor, a glycoprotein that consists of two extracellular α subunits and two β subunits that span the cell membrane. The insulin receptor has tyrosine kinase enzyme activity (residing in the β subunit), which is stimulated when insulin binds to the receptor. This enzyme phosphorylates tyrosine amino acid residues on various intracellular proteins, such as insulin receptor substrate (IRS)-1 and IRS-2, and the β subunit itself (autophosphorylation). Tyrosine kinase activity is essential for insulin action.

FIGURE 5.12

The insulin receptor and its structural domains. Many mutations have been discovered in the insulin receptor, some of which interfere with insulin's action and can cause insulin resistance; examples are shown in the right column.

33

Post-receptor signalling involves phosphorylation of a number of intracellular proteins that associate with the β subunit of the insulin receptor, including IRS-1 and IRS-2. Phosphorylated tyrosine residues on these proteins act as docking sites for the non-covalent binding of proteins with specific 'SH2' domains, such as phospatidylinositol 3-kinase (PI 3-kinase), Grb2 and phosphotyrosine phosphatase (SHP2). Binding of Grb2 to IRS-1 initiates a cascade that eventually activates nuclear transcription factors *via* activation of the protein Ras and mitogen-activated protein (MAP) kinase. IRS–PI 3-kinase binding generates phospholipids that modulate other specific kinases and regulate responses such as glucose transport, and protein and glycogen synthesis.

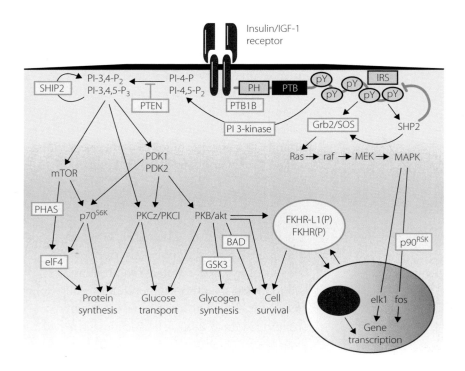

FIGURE 5.13
The insulin signalling cascade. Insulin binding and autophosphorylation of the insulin (and IGF-1) receptor results in binding of the IRS-1 protein to the β subunit of the insulin receptor *via* the IRS phosphotyrosine-binding domain (PTB). There is then phosphorylation of a number of tyrosine residues (pY) at the C-terminus of the IRS proteins. This leads to a recruitment and binding of downstream signalling proteins, such as PI-3 kinase, Grb2 and SHP2

HANDBOOK OF DIABETES 3RD EDITION

After binding of insulin to its receptor, the insulin–receptor complex is internalized by the surrounding membrane invaginating to form an 'endosome'. The protein clathrin plays a key role in the process of endosome formation. After internalization, the receptors are recycled to the cell surface, but insulin is degraded inside the cell by lysosomes. Elevated insulin levels, as in obesity and type 2 diabetes, lead to 'down-regulation' of the receptor, whereby internalization results in decreased receptor numbers at the cell surface.

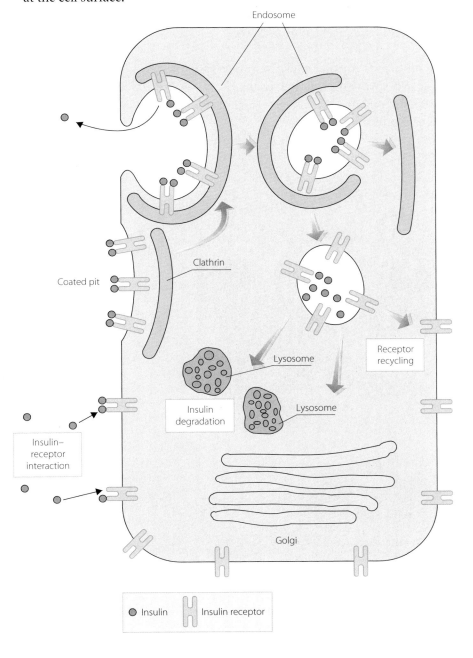

FIGURE 5.14
Insulin receptor internalization.

Glucose is carried across the cell membrane into cells by a family of specialized transporter proteins called glucose transporters (GLUTs). The process is energy independent. The best-characterized GLUTs are:

- GLUT-1, ubiquitously expressed and probably responsible for basal, non-insulin-mediated glucose uptake.
- GLUT-2: present in the islet β cell, and also in the liver, intestine and kidney. Together with glucokinase, it forms the β cell's glucose sensor and, because it has a high K_m, allows glucose to enter the β cell at a rate proportional to the extracellular glucose level.
- GLUT-3: together with GLUT-1, involved in non-insulin-mediated uptake of glucose into the brain.
- GLUT-4: responsible for insulin-stimulated glucose uptake in muscle and adipose tissue, and thus the classic hypoglycaemic action of insulin.
- GLUT-8: important in blastocyst development.
- GLUT-9 and 10: unclear functional significance.

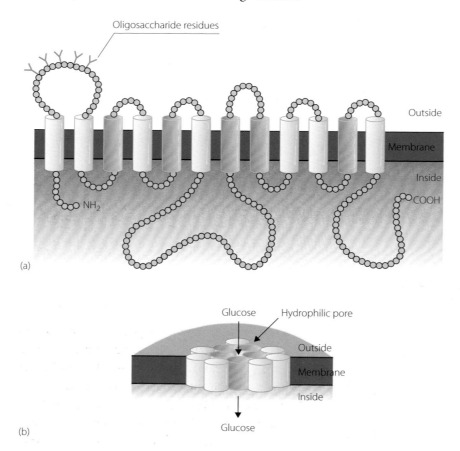

FIGURE 5.15
(a) The structure of a typical GLUT. (b) The intramembrane domains pack together to form a central hydrophilic channel through which glucose passes.

Most of the other GLUTs are present at the cell surface, but in the basal state GLUT-4 is sequestered within vesicles in the cytoplasm. Insulin causes the vesicles to be translocated to the cell surface, where they fuse with the membrane and the inserted GLUT-4 unit functions as a pore that allows glucose entry. The process is reversible: when insulin levels fall, the plasma membrane GLUT-4 is removed by endocytosis and recycled back to vesicles for storage.

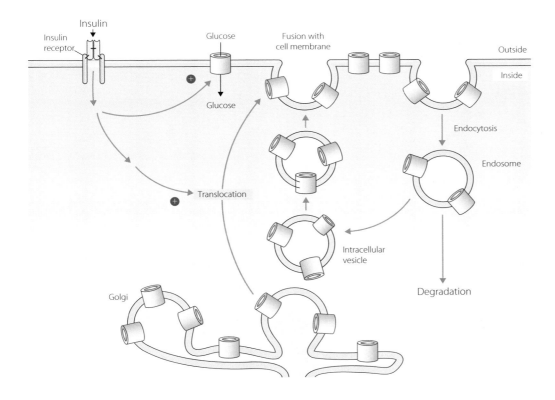

FIGURE 5.16
Insulin regulation of glucose transport into cells.

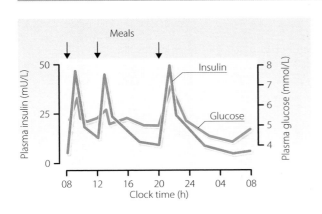

In normal subjects, blood glucose concentrations are maintained within relatively narrow limits at around 5–7 mmol/L (90–126 mg/dL) by the balance between glucose entry into the circulation from the liver and from intestinal absorption, and glucose uptake into the peripheral tissues such as muscle and adipose tissue. Insulin is secreted at a low, basal level, with increased, stimulated levels at mealtimes.

FIGURE 5.17
Profiles of plasma glucose and insulin concentrations in non-diabetic individuals.

At rest in the fasting state, the brain consumes about 80% of the glucose utilized by the whole body, but brain glucose uptake is not regulated by insulin. Glucose is the main fuel for the brain, so that brain function critically depends on the maintenance of normal blood glucose levels.

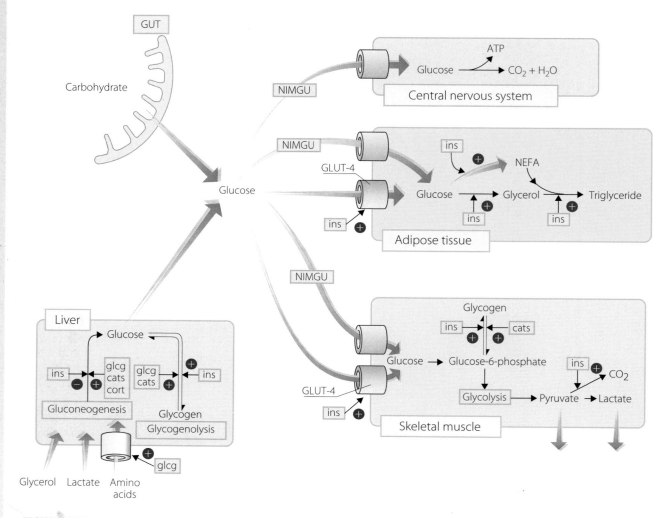

FIGURE 5.18
Overview of carbohydrate metabolism: cats, catecholamines; cort, cortisol; glcg, glucagon; ins, insulin; NIMGU, non-insulin-mediated glucose uptake.

Insulin lowers glucose levels partly by suppressing glucose output from the liver, both by inhibiting glycogen breakdown (glycogenolysis) and by inhibiting gluconeogenesis (i.e. the formation of 'new' glucose from sources such as glycerol, lactate and amino acids, like alanine). Relatively low concentrations of insulin are needed to suppress hepatic glucose output in this way, such as occur with basal insulin secretion between meals and at night. With much higher insulin levels after meals, GLUT-4-mediated glucose uptake into the periphery is stimulated.

EPIDEMIOLOGY AND AETIOLOGY OF TYPE 1 DIABETES

6

The most common cause of type 1 diabetes (over 90% of cases) is T-cell mediated autoimmune destruction of the islet β cells. The exact aetiology is complex and still imperfectly understood. However, it is probable that environmental factors trigger the onset of diabetes in individuals with an inherited predisposition. Unless insulin replacement is given, severe insulin deficiency results in hyperglycaemia and ketoacidosis, the biochemical hallmarks of type 1 diabetes.

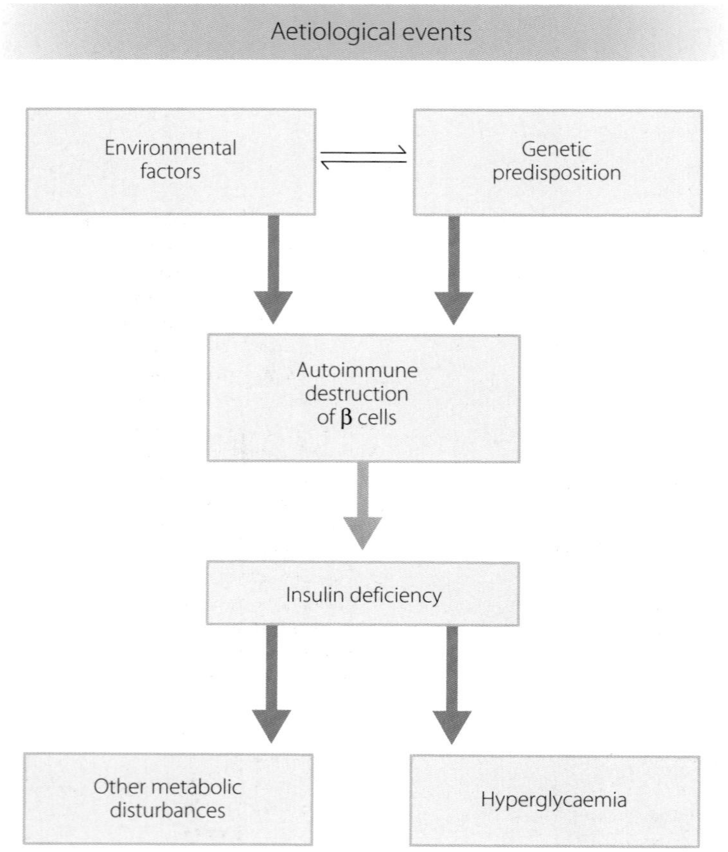

Aetiological events

FIGURE 6.1
Aetiology of type 1 diabetes.

HANDBOOK OF DIABETES 3RD EDITION

There is a striking variation in the incidence of type 1 diabetes between and within populations, with high frequencies in Finland (49 cases/100 000/year) and Sweden (32/100 000/year), and low frequencies in areas of China and Venezuela (both 0.1/100 000/year) and in the Ukraine (1/100 000/year). Marked differences also occur within the same country: the incidence in Sardinia (37/100 000/year) is 3–5 times that of mainland Italy. These differences in frequency suggest that environmental and/or ethnic–genetic factors strongly influence the onset of the disease.

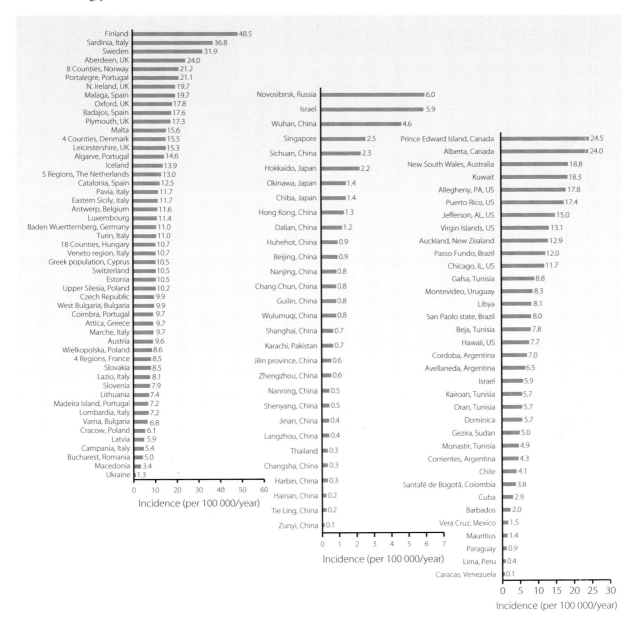

FIGURE 6.2
Age-standardized incidence of type 1 diabetes in children ≤14 years of age (per 100 000 per year).

41

The geographical variation within Europe has been highlighted by the EURODIAB epidemiology study. This survey found a 10-fold difference in the incidence of type 1 diabetes between Finland and Macedonia. The incidence generally falls along a North–South gradient, but Sardinia is a notable 'hot spot', with a much higher frequency than the surrounding Mediterranean areas. Interestingly, there are also different incidences between genetically similar countries such as Finland and Estonia, or Norway and Iceland. This suggests that environmental influences may predominate over genetic susceptibility in causing or triggering the disease.

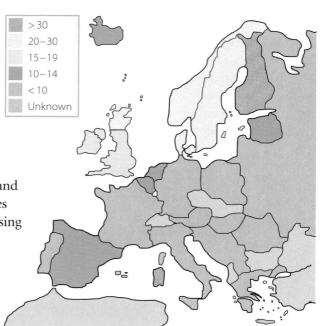

FIGURE 6.3
Incidence rates (cases per 100·000/year) of type 1 diabetes (onset 0–14 years) in Europe. Note the high incidence in Nordic countries, Scotland and Sardinia.

Further evidence for environmental influences comes from studies that show a seasonal variation in the onset of type 1 diabetes in some populations, with the highest frequency in the colder autumn and winter months. This is often thought to reflect seasonal exposure to viruses, but food or chemicals might also be involved. Longer term studies are needed to confirm this finding.

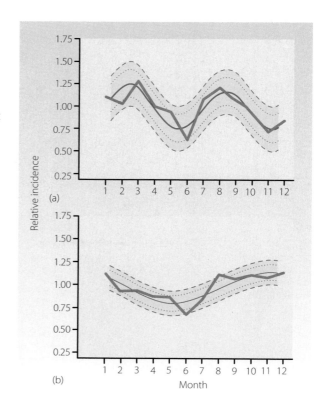

FIGURE 6.4
Seasonal variation of type 1 diabetes among Finnish children during 1983–1992 (a) 0–9 years of age, (b) 10–14 years of age. (The observed monthly variation in incidence is the solid red line.) The inner interval is the 95% confidence interval (CI) for the observed seasonal variation and the outer interval is the 95% CI for the estimated seasonal variation.

HANDBOOK OF DIABETES 3RD EDITION

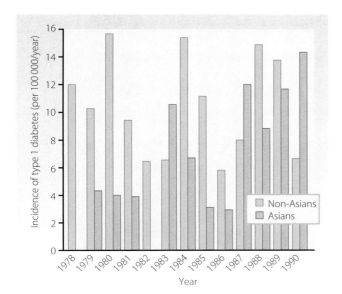

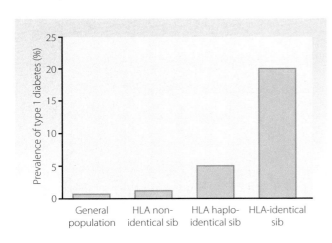

People who have migrated from an area of low incidence for type 1 diabetes to an area of high risk seem to adopt the same level of risk as the population to which they move. For example, children of Asian families (from the Indian subcontinent and Tanzania) who moved to the UK traditionally have a low frequency of type 1 diabetes, but now have a rising incidence of the disease, which is approaching that of the indigenous population.

FIGURE 6.5
Evidence of environmental factors: incidence of type 1 diabetes in children from Asian families who moved to Bradford, UK, compared to non-Asian local UK children.

FIGURE 6.6
Familial clustering of type 1 diabetes: evidence for genetic factors in disease aetiology.

Familial clustering of type 1 diabetes provides evidence for complex genetic factors in its aetiology. In (European) siblings of children with type 1 diabetes, 5–6% have developed type 1 diabetes by the age of 15 years, while 20% develop diabetes if they are human leukocyte antigen (HLA) identical with their diabetic sibling (for comparison, the general population frequency is about 0.4%). However, only 10–15% of type 1 diabetes occurs in families with the disease ('multiplex') and most cases are said to be 'sporadic'.

43

The frequency of type 1 diabetes is increasing in many countries. In Europe, the overall increase is 3.4% per year, but the increase is particularly notable in those diagnosed under the age of 5 years, where it is 6.3% per year. Based on these figures, the incidence of type 1 diabetes may be 40% higher in 2010 than in 1998. This sharp rise in frequency over a short period of time suggests changing environmental factors that operate in early life, rather than any influence of the genetic pattern of the population.

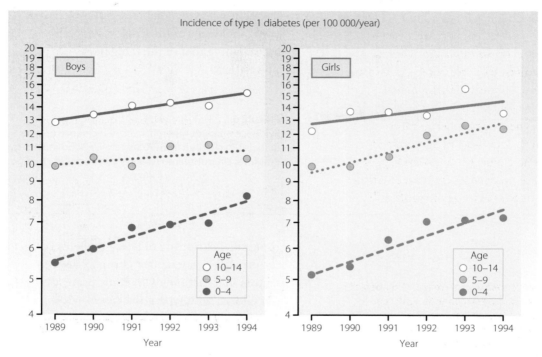

FIGURE 6.7
Trends in childhood diabetes incidence in Europe during 1989–1994 by age and sex.

Evidence for autoimmunity in the pathogenesis of type 1 diabetes includes the presence of a chronic inflammatory mononuclear cell infiltrate ('insulitis') associated with the residual β cells in the islets of recently diagnosed type 1 diabetic patients. The infiltrate consists mainly of T lymphocytes and macrophages. Later in the disease, there is complete loss of β cells, while the other islet cell types (α, δ and PP cells) all survive.

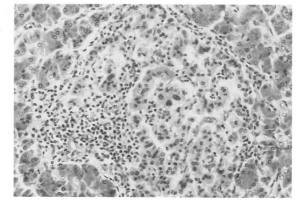

FIGURE 6.8
Insulitis. There is a chronic inflammatory cell infiltrate centred on this islet. Haematoxylin–eosin stain, original magnification ×300.

A major marker of insulitis is the presence in newly diagnosed type 1 diabetic patients of circulating islet-related autoantibodies, such as islet cell autoantibodies (ICAs), insulin autoantibodies (IAAs), IA-2 antibodies and glutamic acid decarboxylase (GAD) autoantibodies. However, not all those with islet autoantibodies develop diabetes, which indicates that insulitis does not necessarily progress to critical β-cell damage. Type 1 diabetes is manifest clinically after a prodromal period of months or years, during which immunological abnormalities, such as circulating islet autoantibodies, can be detected, even though normoglycaemia is maintained. The greatest risk of developing type 1 diabetes is associated with the presence of more than one circulating autoantibody.

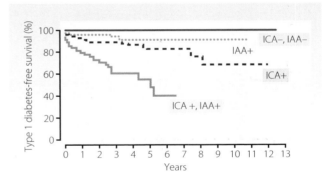

FIGURE 6.9
ICA demonstrated by indirect immunofluorescence in a frozen section of human pancreas.

FIGURE 6.10
The probability of remaining free of type 1 diabetes in 4694 non-diabetic relatives of patients with type 1 diabetes. Susceptibility was dependent on the presence of islet-related antibodies, the greatest risk being when both islet-cell antibodies (ICAs) and insulin autoantibodies (IAAs) were present together.

An autoimmune basis for type 1 diabetes is also suggested by its association with other autoimmune diseases such as hypothyroidism, Graves' disease, pernicious anaemia and Addison's disease.

- Addison's disease
- Graves' disease
- Hypothyroidism
- Hypogonadism
- Pernicious anaemia
- Vitiligo
- Autoimmune polyglandular syndromes, types 1 and 2

FIGURE 6.11
Autoimmune disorders associated with type 1 diabetes.

Genetic susceptibility to type 1 diabetes is most closely associated with HLA genes that lie within the major histocompatibility complex (MHC) region on the short arm of chromosome 6 (this locus is now called *IDDM1*). HLAs are cell-surface glycoproteins that show extreme variability through polymorphisms in the genes that code for them. Over 95% of Caucasian type 1 diabetic subjects carry HLA-DR3 and/or DR4 (class II antigens), as compared with only 50% in non-diabetic individuals.

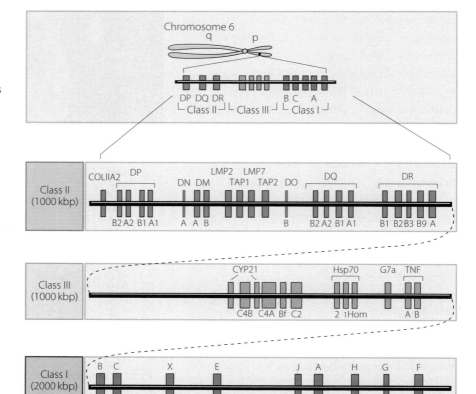

FIGURE 6.12
A simplified map of the MHC region on the short arm of the chromosome (6p21), showing the major genes of classes II, III and I.

Class II HLAs (HLA-D) play a key role in presenting foreign and self-antigens to T- helper lymphocytes and therefore in initiating the autoimmune process. Polymorphisms in the DQB1 gene that result in amino-acid substitutions in the class II antigens may affect the ability to accept and present autoantigens derived from the β cell. This is a critical step in 'arming' T lymphocytes, which initiate the immune attack against the β cells.

FIGURE 6.13
Antigen associated with class II HLA is presented to T cells.

Maximum susceptibility is associated with HLA-DRB1*03.DQ2 and HLA-DRB1*04.DQ8 haplotypes. By contrast, the HLA-DQ6 molecule protects against the disease.

Gene encoding α-chain	Gene encoding β-chain	Corresponding HLA antigen	Effect on diabetes susceptibility
DQA1*0501	DQB1*0201	DQ2	Predisposes
DQA1*0301	DQB1*0302	DQ8	Predisposes
DQA1*0301	DQB1*0301	DQ7	Neutral/protects
DQA1*0102	DQB1*0602	DQ6	Protects
DQA1*0103	DQB1*0603	DQ18	Protects

FIGURE 6.14
Polymorphisms of the *HLA-DQA1* and *-DQB1* genes. These encode the α and β chains of class II antigens, and the resultant HLAs (defined serologically) are shown, together with the effects that they confer on susceptibility to type 1 diabetes in Caucasian populations. Specific polymorphisms are shown as *0501, etc.

Over 20 regions of the human genome are associated with type 1 diabetes, but most make only a minor contribution. *IDDM2* corresponds to the insulin gene locus on chromosome 11, has a smaller effect than *IDDM1* and acts independently. The predisposing polymorphism in the insulin gene and how it influences the disease has yet to be identified. A number of weaker linkages exist, but their nature and importance are unclear.

Name	Chromosomal location	Defined by marker
IDDM1	6p21 (major histocompatibility complex)	HLA-DQB
IDDM2	11p15 (INS)	INS-VNTR
IDDM3	15q26	D15S107
IDDM4	11q13	FGF3
IDDM5	6q25	ESR1
IDDM6	18q21	D18S64
IDDM7	2q31	D2S152
IDDM8	6q27	D6S264
IDDM9	3q21-q25	D3S1576
IDDM10	10p13-q11	D10S193
IDDM11	14q24-q31	D14S67
IDDM12	2q33	CTLA4
IDDM13	2q34	D2S301
IDDM14	Not published	
IDDM15	6q21	D6S283
IDDM16	Not published	
IDDM17	10q25	
IDDM18	5q33–34	IL12B
–	14q12-q21	D14S70-76
–	16q22-q24	D16S515-520
–	19p13	D19S247-226
–	19q13	D19S225
–	1q	D1S1644-AGT
–	Xp13-p11	DX1068

p, q, short, long arms of the numbered chromosome; VNTR, variable number of tandem repeats.

FIGURE 6.15
Loci in the human genome associated with susceptibility to type 1 diabetes.

Much of the evidence that links environmental factors with the aetiology of type 1 diabetes is circumstantial, based on epidemiology and animal research. The factors most often implicated are viruses, diet and toxins, but a number of others, such as breastfeeding and psychological stress, are being investigated.

- Viruses
- Food components and/or toxins:
  N-nitroso compounds
  cow's milk
  wheat proteins
- Psychological stress
- Low exposure to sunlight and/or low vitamin D

FIGURE 6.16
Possible environmental factors that influence the development of type 1 diabetes.

Most viruses have been implicated in human diabetes by temporal and geographical associations between type 1 diabetes and a viral infection. For example, mumps occasionally precedes type 1 diabetes, while intrauterine rubella infection induces diabetes in up to 20% of cases. Many people with recent-onset type 1 diabetes have serological or clinical evidence of Coxsackie B virus infection, particularly the B4 serotype. Marked islet β-cell damage has been detected in children who died from Coxsackie B virus infection.

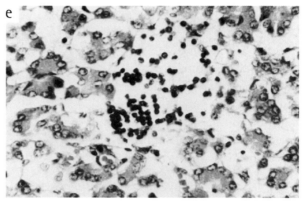

FIGURE 6.17
Histological section of pancreas from a 10-year-old boy infected with Coxsackie B4 virus, who died after the acute onset of type 1 diabetes. The section shows extensive insulitis and severe islet destruction (×160).

In a few cases, Coxsackie viral antigens have been identified in islets *post mortem*, while viruses isolated from the pancreas have been shown to induce diabetes in susceptible mouse strains. Electron microscopy of the pancreas in some subjects who died shortly after the onset of type 1 diabetes has identified retrovirus-like particles within the β cells associated with insulitis.

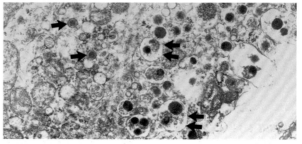

FIGURE 6.18
Retrovirus-like particles (arrows) within damaged β cells from a patient who died with recent-onset type 1 diabetes. Some particles lie within insulin secretory vesicles (double arrows). Electron micrographs, original magnification ×8000.

Viruses may target the β cells and destroy them directly through a cytolytic effect, or by triggering an autoimmune attack against the β cells. Autoimmune mechanisms may include 'molecular mimicry' – i.e. immune responses against a viral antigen that cross-react with a β-cell antigen [e.g. a Coxsackie B4 protein (P2-C) has sequence homology with GAD, an established autoantigen in the β cell]. Also, anti-insulin antibodies from type 1 diabetic patients cross-react with the retroviral p73 antigen in about 75% of cases. Alternatively, viral damage may release sequestered islet antigens and thus restimulate resting autoreactive T cells, previously sensitized against β cell antigens ('bystander activation'). Persistent viral infection could also stimulate interferon-α synthesis and hyperexpression of HLA class I antigens, and the secretion of chemokines that recruit activated macrophages and cytotoxic T cells.

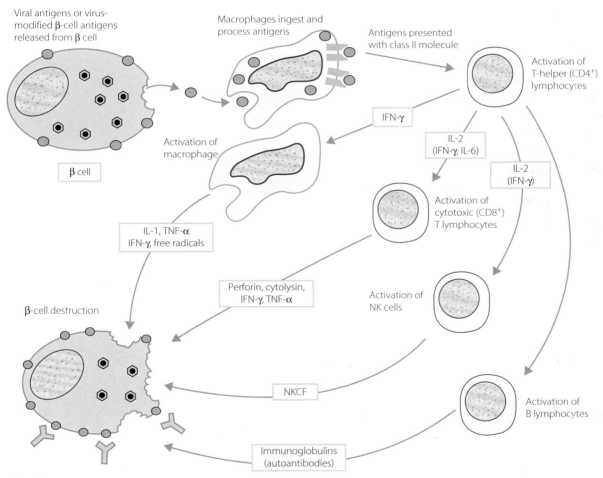

FIGURE 6.19
Hypothetical scheme that shows ways in which viruses could initiate an autoimmune attack on β cells. Some viruses (e.g. retroviruses and rubella virus) may induce β cells to express viral (foreign) antigens, or render an endogenous β-cell antigen immunogenic. Viral antigens released from β cells during normal β-cell turnover might be processed by macrophages and presented to T-helper lymphocytes (CD4⁺) associated with HLA class II antigens. Activated T lymphocytes then secrete interleukin (IL)-2 and other cytokines that activate other immune cells. B lymphocytes produce immunoglobulins against the viral antigens, while activated natural killer (NK) cells and cytotoxic (CD8⁺) lymphocytes cause destruction of β cells that carry the viral antigens. Macrophages, activated by interferon-γ (IFN-γ), also participate in the destruction of the target cells. NKCF, natural killer cell factor; TNF, tumour necrosis factor.

One model of β-cell destruction is via the process of apoptosis, or programmed cell death. This is effected by the activation of cellular caspase enzymes triggered by several means, including the interaction of cell-surface Fas (the death-signalling molecule) with its ligand FasL on the surface of infiltrating cells. Other factors that induce apoptosis include macrophage-derived nitric oxide (NO) and toxic free-radicals, and disruption of the cell membrane by perforin and granzyme B produced by cytotoxic T cells. T-cell cytokines (e.g. interleukin-1, tumour necrosis factor α, interferon-γ) upregulate both Fas and FasL, and also induce NO and toxic free-radicals.

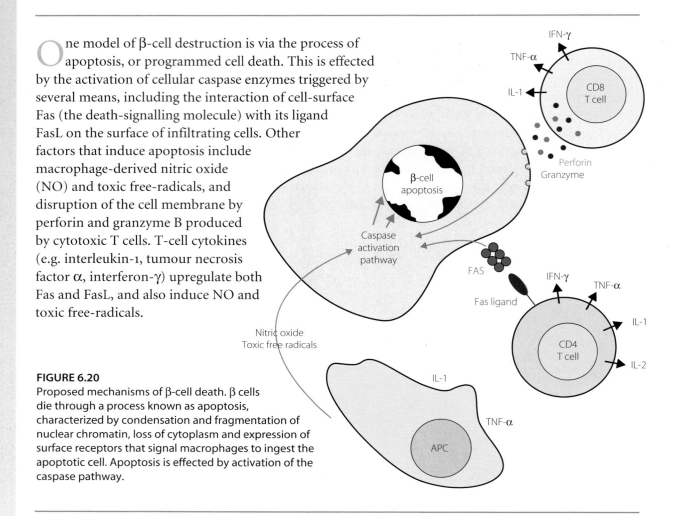

FIGURE 6.20
Proposed mechanisms of β-cell death. β cells die through a process known as apoptosis, characterized by condensation and fragmentation of nuclear chromatin, loss of cytoplasm and expression of surface receptors that signal macrophages to ingest the apoptotic cell. Apoptosis is effected by activation of the caspase pathway.

Wheat gluten is a potent diabetogen in animal models of type 1 diabetes (BB rats and NOD mice, see below), and 5–10% of type 1 diabetic patients have gluten-sensitive enteropathy (coeliac disease). Wheat may induce subclinical gut inflammation and enhanced gut permeability to lumen antigens in some type 1 diabetic patients, which may lead to a breakdown in tolerance for dietary proteins. Other possible diabetogenic factors in diet include *N*-nitroso compounds, speculatively implicated in Icelandic smoked meat.

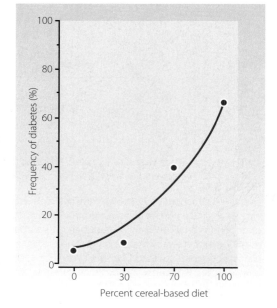

FIGURE 6.21
Increasing the amount of a cereal-based diet (NIH-07) in the food of BB rats from weaning to 140 days increases the percentage of animals that develop type 1 diabetes.

HANDBOOK OF DIABETES 3RD EDITION

It has been suggested that early weaning and introduction of cow's milk may trigger type 1 diabetes, but this remains controversial. Surveys have shown associations between both the consumption of milk protein and a low prevalence of breastfeeding with the incidence of type 1 diabetes in different countries. It is hypothesized that antibodies against bovine serum albumin may cross-react with an islet antigen (ICA69). The studies are inconsistent, perhaps because of variations in milk composition or the existence of a subset of milk-sensitive, diabetes-prone people. Immune tolerance to insulin might also be compromised by cow's milk, which contains much less insulin than human milk.

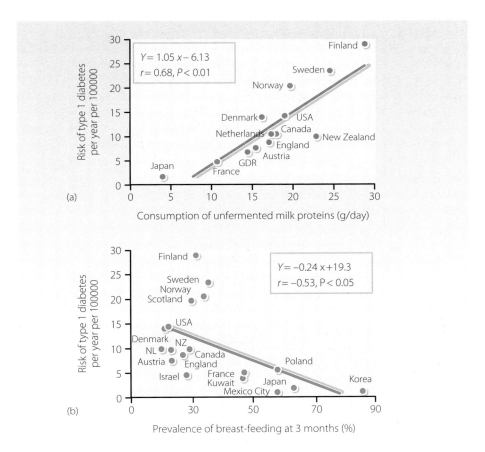

FIGURE 6.22
The relationship between risk of type 1 diabetes and (a) the consumption of milk protein and (b) the prevalence of breast-feeding in different countries.

The notion that there may be environmental β-cell toxins is supported by the existence of chemicals that cause an insulin-dependent type of diabetes in animals. Examples are alloxan and streptozocin, both of which damage the β cell at several sites, including membrane disruption, enzyme inactivation (e.g. glucokinase) and DNA fragmentation. Both drugs are used to induce experimental diabetes in rodents.

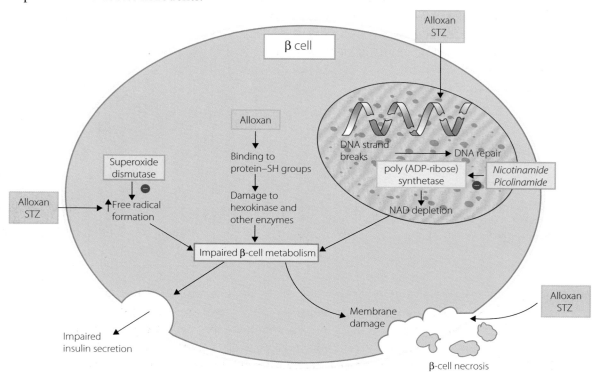

FIGURE 6.23
Suggested mechanisms of alloxan and streptozocin toxicity on the β cell. Inhibitors of poly(ADP-ribose) synthetase, such as nicotinamide and superoxide dismutase (a free-radical scavenger), can protect against the diabetogenic effects of these agents. Multiple low doses of streptozocin can also induce autoimmune β-cell damage.

Spontaneous diabetes that resembles type 1 diabetes in humans occurs in some animals, notably the BioBreeding (BB) rat and the non-obese diabetic (NOD) mouse. These 'animal models' have many of the same characteristics as human autoimmune diabetes, including a genetic predisposition, MHC association, insulitis, circulating islet-cell surface and GAD autoantibodies, a long prediabetic period that precedes overt hyperglycaemia and environmental factors that trigger or accelerate the appearance of diabetes, such as wheat and cow's milk proteins.

(a)

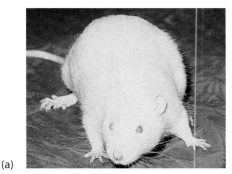

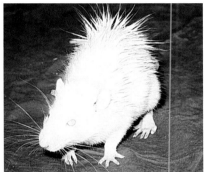

(b)

FIGURE 6.24
A diabetes-prone BB rat (a) before and (b) a few days after the onset of diabetes. Note weight loss and poor grooming (apathy).

One model of the evolution of type 1 diabetes is that individuals destined to develop the disease are born with genes that confer predisposition and outweigh genes with protective effects. Environmental factors act as triggers or that regulators of the T-cell mediated autoimmune destructive process, which results in insulitis, β-cell injury and loss of β-cell mass. As β-cell function declines, there is loss of the first-phase insulin response to intravenous glucose; subsequently, this leads to glucose intolerance (pre-diabetes) and eventually the clinical onset of overt diabetes. At the onset of diabetes, not all β cells have been destroyed and their presence can be identified by the presence of circulating C peptide.

An alternative view is that there is chronic interaction between genetic susceptibility, cumulative exposure to environmental factors and immune regulatory processes, perhaps over the entire period until the loss of all β-cell mass.

These events are assumed to proceed more rapidly in children.

FIGURE 6.25
Schematic evolution of type 1 diabetes.

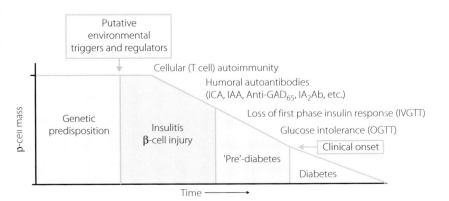

EPIDEMIOLOGY AND AETIOLOGY OF TYPE 2 DIABETES

Type 2 diabetes is the most common type of diabetes, and accounts for about 85% of cases in Caucasian populations. Various clinical risk factors are associated with the disease, such as increasing age, obesity, physical inactivity, a family history of diabetes, and racial and geographical variations in the frequency. These factors give clues to the aetiology and pathophysiology of the disease.

- Race/geographical location
- Age
- Obesity
- Physical inactivity
- Family history of diabetes
- Previous gestational diabetes

FIGURE 7.1
Clinical risk factors for type 2 diabetes.

There is a large variation in the prevalence of type 2 diabetes in different countries. The highest rates are found in some Native American tribes, notably the Pima Indians in Arizona USA (50%), and in the South Pacific Island of Nauru (40%). Low rates are found in poorly developed rural communities, such as parts of Africa (zero in Togo), China and Chile – although rates have risen from <1% to about 3–4% in recent years. The prevalence of impaired glucose tolerance (IGT) tends to decline as the frequency of diabetes increases, which suggests that areas with a high IGT frequency are at an early stage of a diabetes epidemic.

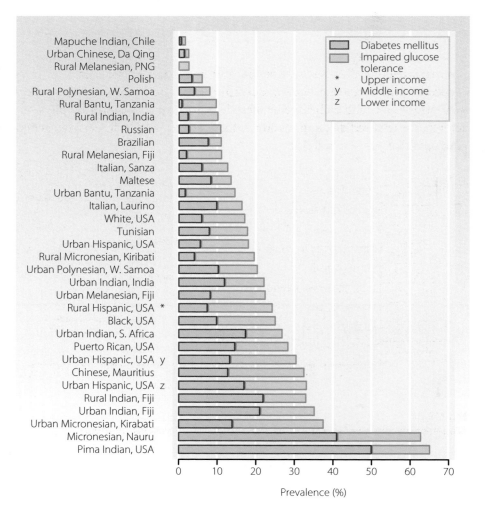

FIGURE 7.2
Prevalence of diabetes and IGT in selected populations in the age range of 30–64 years.

HANDBOOK OF DIABETES 3RD EDITION

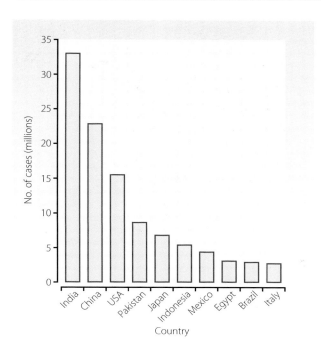

India is now the country with the most diabetic people, and Indian migrants in many parts of the world have a higher frequency of diabetes than the indigenous population has. There has been a progressive rise in the prevalence of diabetes in India since the 1970s, with increases from about 2% to 12% in urban populations. It is estimated that the number of Americans with diabetes will rise from 14 million in 1995 to 22 million in 2025 (overall prevalence >7%), with high rates in US Hispanic people and Black Americans, as well as Native Americans.

FIGURE 7.3
Diabetes around the world. Numbers of cases, adults 20–79 years of age, in selected countries.

In many regions, diabetes is more common in urban than in rural populations. Social deprivation, unemployment and poverty in city dwellers may cosegregate with diabetogenic lifestyle factors, such as decreased physical activity, westernized diet and obesity. Ethnic groups with an underlying genetic predisposition are selected first.

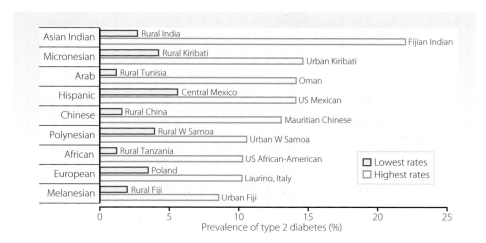

FIGURE 7.4
Diabetes prevalence varies widely between and within different ethnic groups.

The prevalences of type 2 diabetes and IGT increase with age; each affect about 10–20% of subjects over the age of 65 years in many western countries. Most subjects are diagnosed after the age of 40 years, the peak age of onset in developed countries being about 60–70 years.

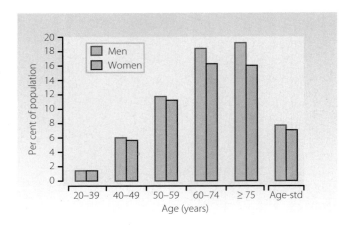

FIGURE 7.5
Prevalence of type 2 diabetes among men and women in the USA. Diabetes was defined as fasting plasma glucose concentration of ≥7.0 mmol/L. Age-std, age-standardized overall prevalence.

In developing countries, the peak age of onset is now 40–45 years – 10–20 years younger than was traditionally the case in the western world. Type 2 diabetes is now starting to present in children and adolescents, usually developing on a background of obesity and a positive family history of diabetes. First reported in susceptible ethnic groups, such as Native Americans, childhood cases are now being reported throughout the world.

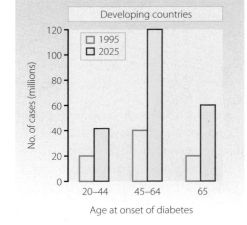

FIGURE 7.6
Age of onset of type 2 diabetes in developing countries. Estimates projected to 2025 suggest that the age at onset will fall progressively.

The important role of obesity in the development of type 2 diabetes is shown by the correlation between the degree of fatness in different countries and the frequency of diabetes.

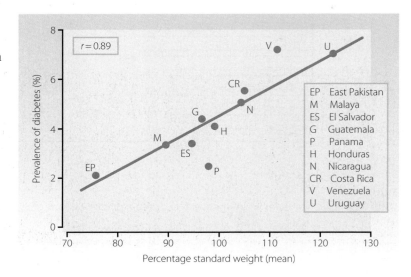

FIGURE 7.7
Diabetes prevalence is closely related to prevalence of obesity.

HANDBOOK OF DIABETES 3RD EDITION

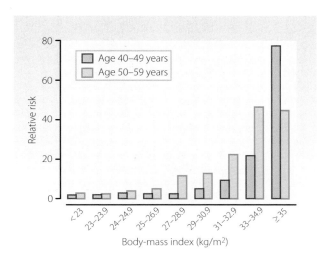

About 80% of type 2 diabetic subjects are obese, and the risk of developing diabetes increases progressively as the body mass index [BMI, weight (kg)/height (m)²] increases. A BMI >35 kg/m² increases the risk of type 2 diabetes developing over a 10-year period by 80-fold, as compared with those with a BMI <22 kg/m². Obesity is still widely defined as a BMI >30 kg/m², though the BMI does not accurately reflect fat mass or its distribution, and is not the best predictor of diabetes.

FIGURE 7.8
Obesity is a risk factor for type 2 diabetes.

The greatest risk of diabetes is associated with central or truncal obesity, in which fat is deposited subcutaneously and at intra-abdominal (visceral) sites. This type of obesity is more typical of men and has therefore been known as 'android' (cf. gluteofemoral or 'gynoid' obesity, more typical of women). In clinical practice, central obesity can be assessed by the weight:hip circumference ratio, but simple measurements of waist circumference are also useful, especially in predicting cardiovascular risk. In obesity, fat also accumulates at other sites (notably within muscle, liver and islet cells) and may contribute to metabolic defects, such as insulin resistance.

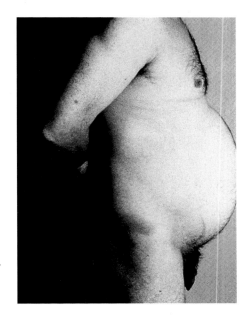

FIGURE 7.9
Central obesity in a man.

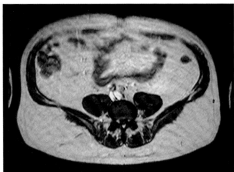
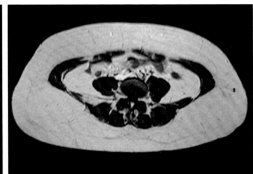

FIGURE 7.10
Magnetic resonance scans showing (a) central and (b) gluteofemoral obesity.

(a)　　　　(b)　　　　59

Obesity contributes to diabetes by causing insulin resistance, the best relationship being with the amount of visceral fat.

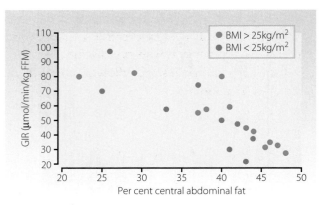

FIGURE 7.11
Insulin resistance (GIR) is proportional to visceral fat mass, independent of BMI. FFM, fat-free mass; GIR, glucose infusion rate.

Visceral fat liberates large amounts of non-esterified fatty acids (NEFAs) through lipolysis, which increase gluoconeogenesis in the liver and impair glucose uptake and utilization in muscle. NEFAs may also inhibit insulin secretion, possibly by enhancing the accumulation of triglyceride within the β cells. In addition, adipose tissue produces cytokines, such as tumour necrosis factor (TNF) α, resistin and IL-6, which experimentally interfere with insulin action. There is often increased sympathetic nervous system activity in obesity, which might also increase lipolysis, reduce muscle blood flow (and thus glucose delivery) and directly affect insulin action.

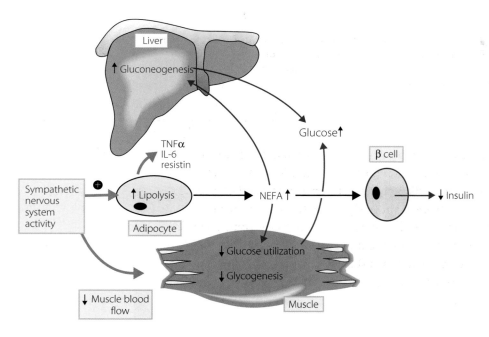

FIGURE 7.12
Mechanisms of insulin resistance in type 2 diabetes.

HANDBOOK OF DIABETES 3RD EDITION

Low levels of physical exercise also predict the development of type 2 diabetes, possibly because exercise both increases insulin sensitivity and prevents obesity. Subjects who exercise the most have a 25–60% lower risk of developing type 2 diabetes, regardless of other risk factors, such as obesity and family history of diabetes.

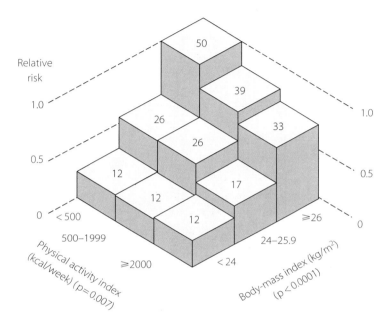

FIGURE 7.13
Age-adjusted risk of type 2 diabetes among 5990 men. The figure shows data for the physical activity index in relation to BMI. Each block represents the relative risk of type 2 diabetes per 10·000 man-years of follow-up, with the risk for the tallest block set at 1.0. The numbers on the blocks are incidence rates of type 2 diabetes per 10·000 man-years.

Evidence for a genetic basis to type 2 diabetes includes that it shows clear familial aggregation, but it does not segregate in a classic Mendelian fashion. About 10% of patients with type 2 diabetes have a similarly affected sibling. The concordance rate for identical twins is variously estimated to be 33–90% (17–37% in non-identical twins), but the interpretation of this is controversial. Part of the explanation for the high concordance may be non-genetic, in that these twins usually share a single placenta and are influenced by the same intrauterine environment (see below).

Unlike type 1 diabetes, type 2 diabetes is not associated with genes in the HLA region – it is probably multigenic with many different combinations of possible gene defects. Candidate genes tested and identified as having an association in some families include the insulin promoter, some transcription factors such as hepatic nuclear factor 4A, peroxisome proliferator-activated receptor-γ and insulin receptor substrate-1. To date, however, no genes have been identified that have a moderate or major effect on the disease. In genome-wide scans of diabetic families, loci for type 2 diabetes have been found at several sites in different populations. The chromosome 2q (*NIDDM1*) locus, for example, codes for calpain 10, a protease of uncertain function.

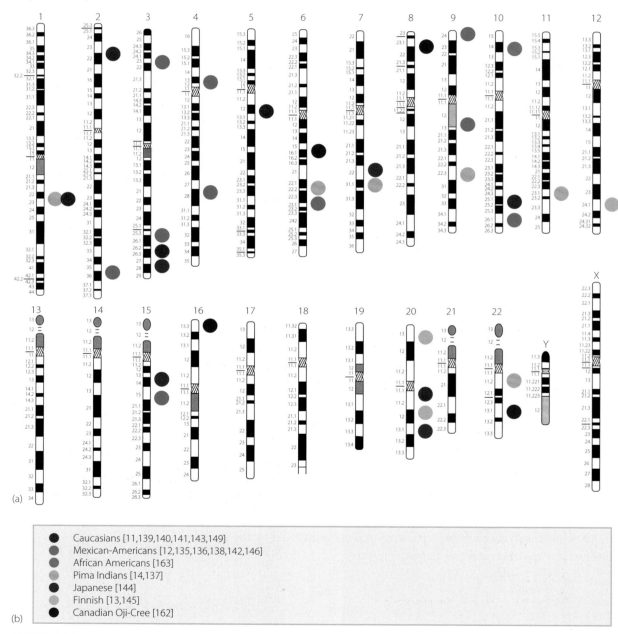

FIGURE 7.14
Type 2 diabetes loci identified in genome-wide scan studies. (a) Chromosomal locations. (b) Positive linkage with type 2 diabetes and related phenotypes in different populations.

HANDBOOK OF DIABETES 3RD EDITION

An influence of intrauterine and neonatal nutrition on the later development of type 2 diabetes was first suggested by a study of a cohort of men born in 1920–1930 in Hertfordshire, UK. Those with a low birthweight had the highest frequency of diabetes and IGT in adult life. It has been proposed that fetal and early childhood malnutrition programmes metabolism by impairing β-cell development and inducing insulin resistance. If nutrition is abundant in adult life, leading to obesity, then IGT and diabetes result. This has been called the 'thrifty phenotype' hypothesis. Further studies have shown that coronary heart disease, hypertension and dyslipidaemia (metabolic syndrome X, see below) are also associated with low birthweight.

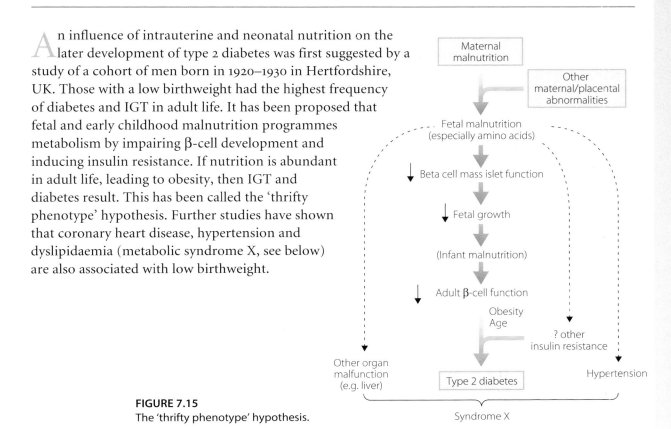

FIGURE 7.15
The 'thrifty phenotype' hypothesis.

Type 2 diabetes develops because of a progressive deterioration of β-cell function, coupled with increasing insulin resistance for which the β cell cannot compensate. At the time of diagnosis, β-cell function is already reduced by about 50% and continues to decline, regardless of therapy.

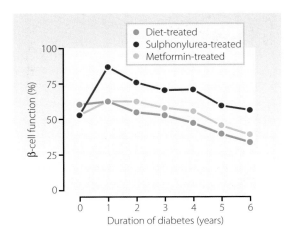

FIGURE 7.16
β-cell function as measured by the homeostasis model assessment (HOMA) method (calculated from the fasting blood glucose and insulin concentrations) in type 2 diabetic patients from the UK Prospective Diabetes Study (UKPDS). β-cell function is already reduced to 50% at diagnosis and declines thereafter, despite therapy.

The main defects in β-cell function in type 2 diabetes include markedly reduced first- and second-phase insulin responses to intravenous glucose, and delayed or blunted responses to mixed meals. There are also alterations in pulsatile and ultradian oscillations of insulin release and increases in the proportions of plasma proinsulin and split proinsulin peptides relative to insulin. Most of these abnormalities are present in IGT, and some in normoglycaemic first-degree relatives or the monozygotic twin of people with type 2 diabetes. This indicates that impaired β-cell function is an early, possibly genetic, defect in the natural history of type 2 diabetes.

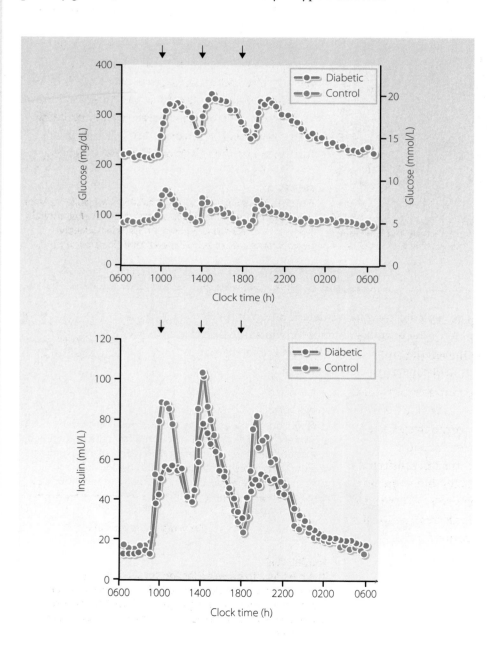

FIGURE 7.17
Plasma concentrations of glucose and insulin in type 2 diabetic and non-diabetic control subjects in response to mixed meals

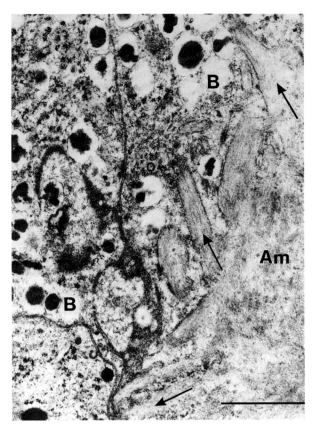

The main histological abnormality in the islets of type 2 diabetic patients (>90%) is the presence of amyloid, insoluble fibrils that lie outside the cells and derive from islet amyloid polypeptide (IAPP; also known as amylin). IAPP is co-secreted with insulin in a molar ratio of 1:10–50. Although IAPP is reported to impair insulin secretion and to be toxic to the β-cell, it is thought unlikely to play a major role in the pathogenesis of type 2 diabetes: for example, islet amyloid deposits are found in up to 20% of elderly people with normal glucose tolerance. The β-cell mass is decreased by only 20–40% in type 2 diabetes – which cannot explain the >80% reduction in insulin release. Additional functional defects in the β cell present in established diabetes may include glucotoxicity and lipotoxicity (i.e. toxic effects of glucose and NEFAs on β-cell function) and the effects of IAPP oversecretion.

FIGURE 7.18
Electron micrographic appearances of islet amyloid deposits in type 2 diabetes. In a patient with type 2 diabetes, amyloid (Am) fibrils closely surround the β cells (B) and deeply invaginate the distorted cell membrane. Scale bar, 1 μm.

Resistance to the biological effects of insulin can be demonstrated in type 2 diabetes by several methods including the euglycaemic hyperinsulinaemic clamp, in which a fixed amount of insulin is infused intravenously and a titrated infusion of intravenous glucose is administered to maintain normoglycaemia. A low rate of exogenous glucose infusion indicates insulin resistance. Insulin sensitivity is generally low in type 2 diabetes, but some non-diabetic people are as insulin resistant as those with type 2 diabetes. This indicates that insulin resistance alone cannot account for the development of diabetes.

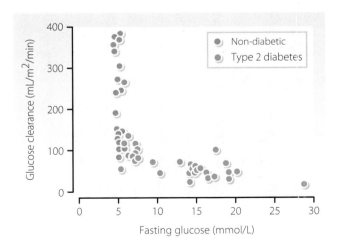

FIGURE 7.19
The relationship between fasting plasma glucose concentration and glucose metabolic clearance rates (insulin sensitivity) observed during hyperinsulinaemic, glucose-clamp studies in non-diabetic subjects and patients with type 2 diabetes.

Insulin resistance is often associated with a clustering of clinical and biochemical features, known as 'metabolic syndrome X' or the 'insulin resistance' syndrome. This consists of glucose intolerance (type 2 diabetes or IGT), central obesity, hypertension, accelerated atherosclerosis, low serum high-density lipoprotein (HDL) cholesterol and high triglyceride/very low-density lipoprotein (VLDL) concentrations. This lipid abnormality of low HDL and high triglyceride is characteristic of type 2 diabetes (and not type 1 diabetes), and is known as 'diabetic dyslipidaemia' (see Chapter 18). Other abnormalities associated with the insulin resistance syndrome are increased concentrations of procoagulant factors, such as plasminogen activator inhibitor-1 (PAI-1) and fibrinogen, which may play a role in promoting atheroma formation.

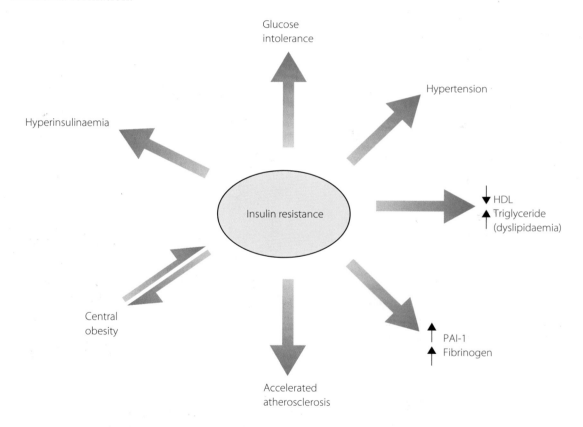

FIGURE 7.20
The 'insulin resistance syndrome' (metabolic syndrome X).

HANDBOOK OF DIABETES *3RD EDITION*

Various neuroendocrine peptides and cytokines play roles in some genetic type 2 diabetes-like syndromes in animals; their roles in the human disease are probably minimal. Leptin is a protein secreted by adipose tissue that inhibits feeding in rodents, possibly by inhibiting neuropeptide Y neurones (which stimulate feeding) in the hypothalamus. Leptin defects give rise to overeating and obesity in rodents; mutations in the leptin gene are present in the genetically obese diabetic *ob/ob* mouse, and mutations in the hypothalamic leptin receptor occur in the diabetic, obese and insulin resistant *db/db* mouse and *fa/fa* rat. Although there are very rare mutations of leptin and its receptor in humans, the role of leptin in common type 2 diabetes is unclear. Adipose tissue also secretes the cytokine TNFα, which may cause insulin resistance by inhibiting the tyrosine kinase activity of the insulin receptor and decreasing the expression of the glucose transporter, GLUT-4. IL-6, secreted by adipose tissue and other cells, also induces insulin resistance. The protein adiponectin is secreted by fat cells and ameliorates insulin resistance, probably by increasing fat oxidation; circulating levels are low in human obesity. The role of the protein resistin, also secreted by adipocytes and implicated in insulin resistance, needs clarifying.

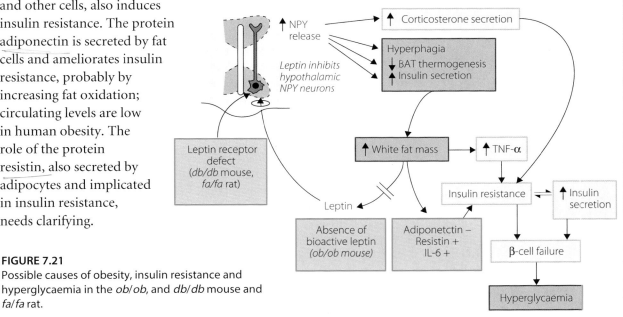

FIGURE 7.21
Possible causes of obesity, insulin resistance and hyperglycaemia in the *ob/ob*, and *db/db* mouse and *fa/fa* rat.

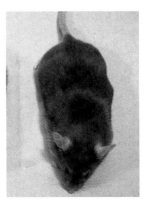

(a)   (b)

FIGURE 7.22
An (a) obese (*ob/ob*) Aston mouse with (b) a lean (+/+) littermate. Obesity (and severe insulin resistance) develop as a result of hyperphagia and reduced energy expenditure, which are caused by the absence of biologically active leptin. This evolves into a hyperglycaemic syndrome that broadly resembles human type 2 diabetes.

Recently, it has been shown that type 2 diabetes is associated with elevated circulating markers of the acute-phase response (part of the innate immune system), such as C-reactive protein and sialic acid. Increased blood levels of these markers and of IL-6 (the major cytokine mediator of the acute-phase response) in non-diabetic subjects predict the later development of type 2 diabetes. Since dyslipidaemia is an acute-phase response and there are mechanisms by which cytokines can cause insulin resistance and features of the metabolic syndrome, it has been hypothesized that activated innate immunity or chronic low-grade inflammation may play a key role in the pathogenesis of type 2 diabetes. Inflammation is also involved in the pathogenesis of atherosclerosis, and activated innate immunity may be the common antecedent of both type 2 diabetes and atherosclerosis.

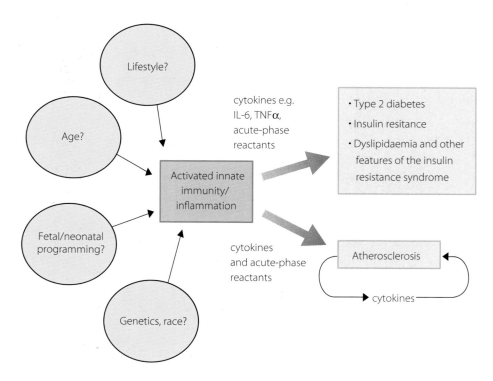

FIGURE 7.23
Chronic low-grade inflammation (activated innate immunity) may be involved in the pathogenesis of type 2 diabetes and atherosclerosis.

Both insulin resistance and β-cell dysfunction are early features of glucose intolerance, and there has been much debate as to whether one is the primary defect and precedes the other during the evolution of type 2 diabetes. In fact, the contributions of insulin resistance and β-cell dysfunction vary considerably among patients, as well as during the course of the disease. Usually, there is a decline in both insulin action and insulin secretion in those who progress from normal glucose tolerance to IGT and diabetes. Both environmental and genetic factors contribute to both insulin resistance and β-cell failure.

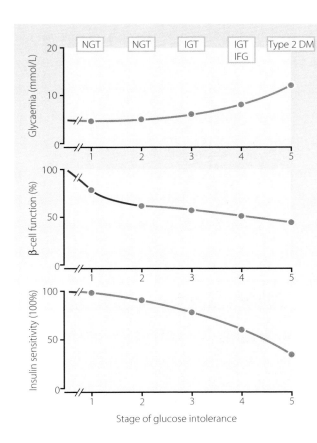

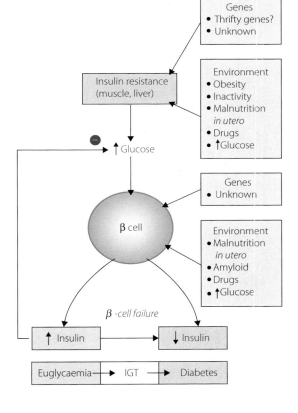

FIGURE 7.24
The stages of glucose tolerance and associated β-cell function and insulin sensitivity, from normal glucose tolerance (NGT) through impaired glucose tolerance (IGT), with or without impaired fasting glucose (IFG), and finally type 2 diabetes mellitus (DM).

FIGURE 7.25
Pathogenesis of type 2 diabetes. Both genetic and environmental factors contribute to both insulin resistance and β-cell failure.

OTHER TYPES OF DIABETES 8

Maturity-onset diabetes of the young (MODY) is a group of non-insulin-dependent diabetic syndromes, defined by early-onset (usually before the age of 25 years), and autosomal inheritance. There is β-cell dysfunction, but in contrast to type 2 diabetes, obesity and/or insulin resistance are rare. MODY accounts for about 1% of diabetic patients in most Caucasian populations. A number of diagnostic criteria help to decide whether a diabetic patient has MODY.

1 Early diagnosis of diabetes – before age 25 years in at least one and ideally two family members

2 Not insulin-dependent – shown by absence of insulin treatment 5 years after diagnosis or significant C-peptide in a patient on insulin treatment

3 Autosomal dominant inheritance, i.e. vertical transmission of diabetes through at least two generations (ideally three generations), with a similar phenotype in cousins or second cousins

4 Rarely obese (obesity is not required for the development of diabetes)

5 Diabetes results from β-cell dysfunction (insulin levels are often in the normal range, though inappropriately low for the degree of hyperglycaemia)

FIGURE 8.1
Diagnostic criteria for maturity-onset diabetes of the young (MODY).

The most common causes of MODY are mutations in either transcription factors (about 75% of cases) or the enzyme glucokinase (about 15%); further MODY genes remain to be identified. Glucokinase MODY (*MODY2*) was the first gene defect shown to cause a non-insulin-dependent type of diabetes. The enzyme is the rate-limiting step in glucose metabolism in the β cell and acts as the β-cell 'glucose sensor' (see Chapter 5). Over 100 different glucokinase mutations have been described. The clinical phenotype is one of mild, stable fasting (not usually post-load) hyperglycaemia, which occurs from birth. It is treated with diet, and tissue complications are rare because hyperglycaemia is mild.

FIGURE 8.2
The different genetic aetiology in a UK maturity-onset diabetes of the young (MODY) series of 132 families. MODYx, clinical MODY where known genes have been excluded; HNF, hepatocyte nuclear factor; IPF, insulin promoter factor.

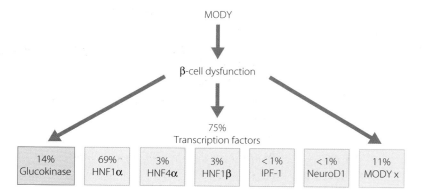

The transcription-factor mutations result in a progressive and frequently severe β-cell defect, often with microvascular complications. The most common type is hepatic nuclear factor-1α (encoded by *HNF1A; MODY3*). Subjects develop diabetes at 10–30 years of age. In contrast to glucokinase MODY, there is marked post-load hyperglycaemia during the oral glucose tolerance test. About one-third are treated by oral hypoglycaemic agents (initially, low doses of a sulphonylurea; there is little response to metformin), and one-third by insulin.

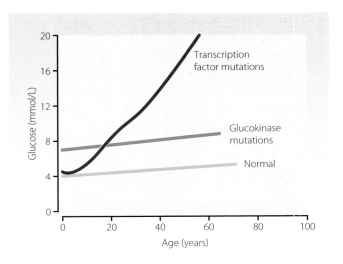

FIGURE 8.3
Variation of blood glucose concentration with age in maturity-onset diabetes of the young (MODY) patients with glucokinase mutations and transcription-factor mutations (most frequently of *HNF1A*).

The differential diagnosis of transcription-factor MODY can be assisted by a variety of extrapancreatic clinical features, such as glycosuria and a raised HDL in mutations of *HNF1A* (MODY3), low triglycerides in *HNF4A* (MODY1), and cystic renal disease and uterine abnormalities in *HNF1B* (MODY5).

Transcription factor	Extrapancreatic clinical features
HNF1A (MODY3)	Low renal threshold (glycosuria)
	Sensitivity to insulin
	Raised HDL
HNF4A (MODY1)	Low fasting triglycerides
	Reduced apolipoproteins apoAII and apoCIII
HNF1B (MODY5)	Renal cysts
	Renal histology includes: glomerulocystic kidney disease, renal dysplasia, oligomeganephronia
	Renal impairment
	Uterine and genital abnormalities
	Hyperuricaemia
	Short stature
IPF-1 (MODY4)	Pancreatic agenesis with homozygote mutations
NEUROD1 (MODY6)	None described

FIGURE 8.4
Extrapancreatic features that help to differentiate various forms of transcription-factor maturity-onset diabetes of the young (MODY).

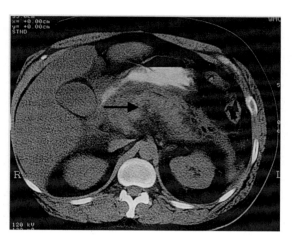

FIGURE 8.5
Acute pancreatitis. Magnetic resonance scan of the abdomen, showing marked oedema and swelling of the gland. Subsequently, a pancreatic pseudocyst developed.

Many pancreatic diseases can cause diabetes, but in total account for <1% of all cases of diabetes. Acute pancreatitis (commonly caused by alcoholism or gallstones) usually results in transient hyperglycaemia, but permanent diabetes occurs in up to 15% of patients. There are usually, but not always, elevated serum amylase and lipase levels, and oedema and swelling of the gland detectable on magnetic resonance or computed tomography imaging.

Chronic pancreatitis, commonly caused by alcoholism in Western countries, leads to IGT or diabetes in 40–50% of cases. Intraductal protein plugs subsequently calcify as the characteristic calcite stones, with cyst formation, inflammation and fibrosis. One-third require insulin, but ketoacidosis is rare. Tropical calcific pancreatitis is confined to India and developing nations, and results in diabetes in 90% of cases ('fibrocalculous pancreatic diabetes'). Even in these countries, it accounts for only 1% of diabetes cases. It is often associated with malnutrition, but the aetiology is not understood. Very large pancreatic stones and steatorrhoea are characteristic. Most patients require insulin.

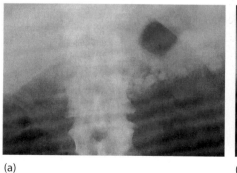
(a)

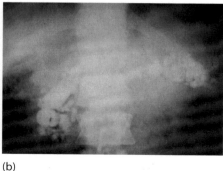
(b)

FIGURE 8.6
Pancreatic calculi, showing characteristic patterns in alcoholic chronic pancreatitis (a), and fibrocalculous pancreatic diabetes (b).

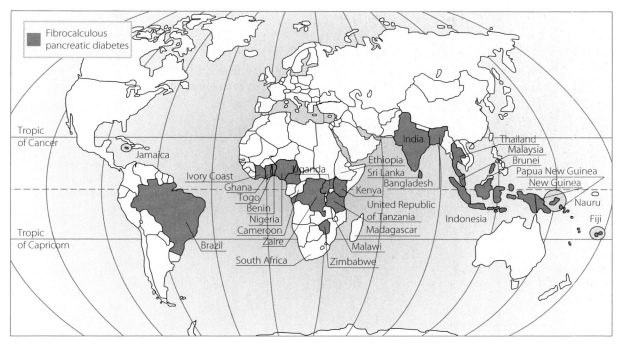

FIGURE 8.7
Worldwide distribution of fibrocalculous pancreatic diabetes. The disease is
confined to tropical and subtropical zones.

Genetic or primary haemochromatosis is an autosomal recessive inborn error of metabolism, usually caused by a mutation in the haemochromatosis gene, *HFE*, on chromosome 6. The HFE protein is expressed on duodenal enterocytes and modulates iron uptake. Haemochromatosis is associated with increased iron absorption and tissue deposition of iron, notably in the liver, islets, skin and pituitary gonadotrophs. The classic triad is hepatic cirrhosis, glucose intolerance (with insulin-requiring diabetes in 25%) and skin hyperpigmentation ('bronzed diabetes'). Serum iron and ferritin concentrations are raised. Secondary haemochromatosis can occur in patients who require frequent blood transfusions (e.g. for β-thalassaemia).

FIGURE 8.8
Bronzing of the skin in a patient with hereditary haemochromatosis.

Pancreatic carcinoma is associated with type 2 diabetes. The diagnosis should be suspected in type 2 patients with unexplained weight loss or back pain. The nature of the association between pancreatic cancer and diabetes is controversial, but diabetes may improve after removal of the tumour. Pancreatic cancer has a very poor prognosis and is increasing in incidence.

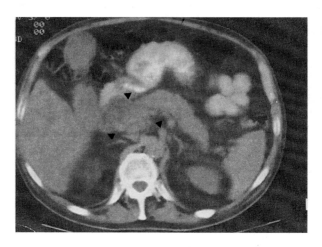

FIGURE 8.9
Carcinoma of the pancreas. This 65-year-old man presented with back pain and obstructive jaundice and was found to have type 2 diabetes. The computed tomography scan shows a mass in the head of the pancreas (arrows) that has obstructed the common bile duct and caused massive dilatation of the intrahepatic bile ducts.

There are several rare genetic and acquired syndromes of severe insulin resistance. Patients often present with marked postprandial hyperglycaemia but normal fasting blood glucose concentrations. Clinical features often seen in these conditions are acanthosis nigricans and hyperandrogenism, both probably a result of compensatory hyperinsulinaemia on tissues and organs. Acanthosis nigricans comprises areas of hyperpigmented, velvety skin, usually in flexures of the axillae, the back of the neck or groin. Hyperandrogenism is common in postpubertal girls with these syndromes, and is manifested as amenorrhoea and/or oligomenorrhoea, hirsutism, acne and polycystic ovaries. An example is 'type A insulin resistance', which almost always affects adolescent females. In 25%, there is a mutation of the tyrosine kinase domain of the β subunit of the insulin receptor.

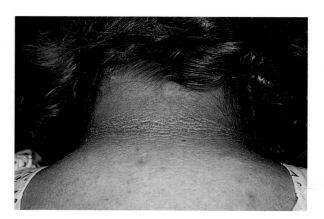

FIGURE 8.10
Acanthosis nigricans on the nape of the neck of a 26-year-old woman with the type A insulin resistance syndrome.

Leprechaunism (Donohue's syndrome) is a rare congenital condition in which there is severe intrauterine and postnatal growth retardation. Patients have dysmorphic facies, acanthosis nigricans, little subcutaneous fat and severe insulin resistance. Mutations affect both alleles of the insulin receptor's α subunit, which results in complete loss of receptor function. Death usually follows in childhood. Rabson–Mendenhall syndrome is also associated with α-subunit insulin-receptor mutations, but only partial loss of receptor function; there is less severe insulin resistance, but frank diabetes occurs.

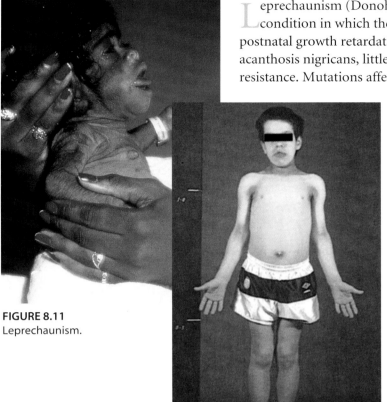

FIGURE 8.11
Leprechaunism.

FIGURE 8.12
Rabson–Mendenhall syndrome in a 13-year-old boy, showing growth retardation, prominent acanthosis nigricans affecting the axillae, neck and antecubital fossae, and typical facies.

Type B insulin resistance is an acquired condition caused by immunoglobulin G (IgG) autoantibodies to the insulin receptor. Patients (who are mostly female) often show manifestations of autoimmune disease, including arthritis, nephritis, vitiligo, alopecia areata and systemic lupus erythematosus. Sometimes there is fluctuating hyper- and hypoglycaemia, as antibodies can be stimulatory or inhibitory at the insulin receptor.

FIGURE 8.13
Type B syndrome of insulin resistance caused by insulin receptor antibodies.

β cell

↑ Insulin

Insulin receptor antibodies

Effects of hyperinsulinaemia

● Acanthosis nigricans
● Polycystic ovaries and hyperandrogenism

Insulin receptor

Impaired insulin action

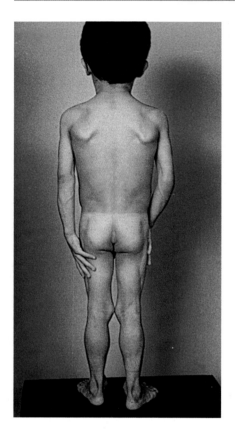

A number of congenital and acquired lipodystrophies are linked with severe insulin resistance. For example, Berardinelli–Seip congenital lipodystrophy (BSCL) is an autosomal-recessive inherited condition with generalized absence of the metabolically active subcutaneous and visceral fat, together with hepatomegaly and acromegalic features. Leptin deficiency, because of lack of the fat that produces it, leads to a voracious appetite. Biochemically, there is glucose intolerance and severe hypertriglyceridaemia. It is genetically heterogeneous, with at least three genes involved in different cases.

FIGURE 8.14
Congenital generalized lipodystrophy (Berardinelli–Seip syndrome). This 7-year-old boy shows apparent total lipoatrophy despite adequate nutrition.

Diabetes or IGT is associated with several syndromes in which there are mutations in mitochondrial DNA (mtDNA), which is inherited maternally. This leads to impaired oxidative phosphorylation and β-cell dysfunction. The main clinical features of these syndromes include neurological abnormalities. For example, a point mutation in mtDNA that encodes the transfer RNA for the amino acid leucine leads to maternally transmitted diabetes with sensorineural deafness, and/or MELAS syndrome (myopathy, encephalopathy, lactic acidosis and stroke-like episodes).

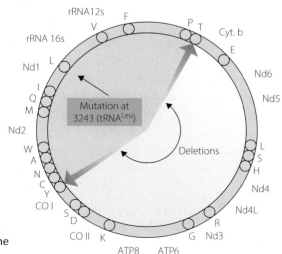

FIGURE 8.15
Structure of the mitochondrial genome. Circles indicate the 22 tRNA genes. The mutation at base pair 3243 is located in the gene for tRNA^{Leu} (arrow).

Wolfram syndrome or DIDMOAD (diabetes insipidus, diabetes mellitus, optic atrophy and deafness) results from both mtDNA mutations and a nuclear gene defect on chromosome 4. Diabetes mellitus usually appears first, in childhood or early adult life, and the other features develop over several years in variable sequence.

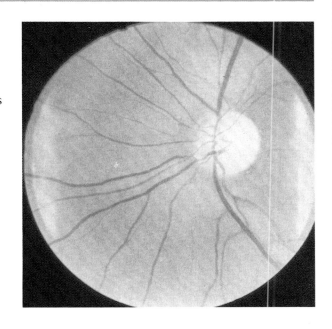

FIGURE 8.16
Optic atrophy, in a patient with Wolfram syndrome (DIDMOAD).

Insulinopathies are rare mutations in the human preproinsulin gene that lead to either incompletely cleaved proinsulin with C peptide still attached or a mutant insulin with diminished bioactivity. Since the individuals are heterozygous, both normal and abnormal insulin are present in the circulation.

Patients with insulinopathies display hyperproinsulinaemia or hyperinsulinaemia, varying degrees of glucose intolerance from normal to diabetes, and a normal response to exogenous insulin. Glucose tolerance of affected subjects deteriorates with age, and non-insulin-dependent diabetes presumably develops following the superimposition of environmental and other genetic factors (not affecting insulin) on the effects of the mutant insulin gene.

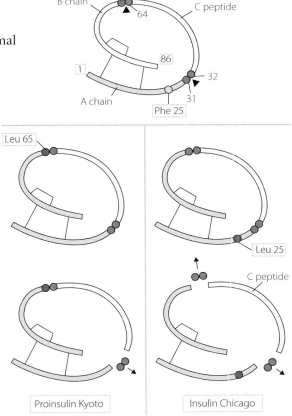

FIGURE 8.17
Molecular basis of insulinopathies. The structure of wild-type proinsulin is indicated at the top. *Left:* Mutations that affect a cleavage site for proteolytic processing enzymes (arrowheads) result in an incompletely processed product of proinsulin (e.g. proinsulin Kyoto). *Right:* Point mutations within the coding regions of the A or B chains produce a mutant insulin, which is normally processed, but may have altered biological activity.

Several endocrine conditions are associated with diabetes mellitus. Cushing's syndrome comprises glucocorticoid excess of any cause, including steroid drug-induced, pituitary adenoma, adrenal tumour, and ectopic ACTH production. Glucocorticoids cause insulin resistance, which stimulates hepatic gluconeogenesis, adipose tissue lipolysis and NEFA release, and inhibits peripheral glucose uptake. Most patients have some degree of glucose intolerance; overt diabetes, usually non-insulin-dependent, but insulin-requiring, affects about 10–20% of cases.

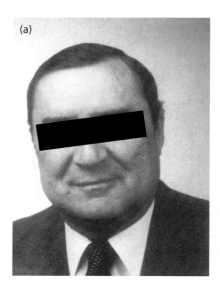

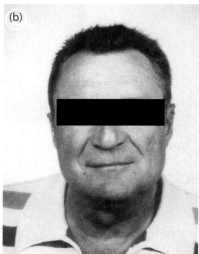

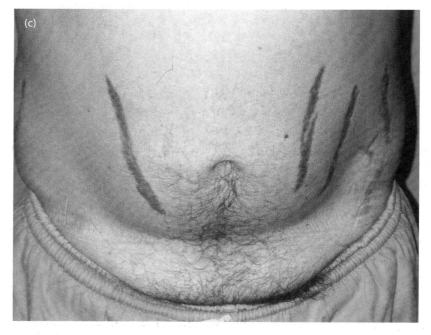

FIGURE 8.18
Cushing's syndrome in a 53-year-old hypertensive man who presented with diabetes that required insulin to control hyperglycaemia. Features included 'moon face' (a) and truncal obesity with reddish-purple striae (c). After removal of the 10-mm corticotroph pituitary adenoma, his facial appearance returned to normal (b), as did his blood pressure and blood glucose.

Acromegaly, i.e. growth hormone excess that results from an anterior pituitary (somatotroph) tumour, causes glucose intolerance by inducing insulin resistance. Overt diabetes (type 2-like)and IGT each affect about one-third of acromegalic patients. As in type 2 diabetes, it has been hypothesized that hyperglycaemia caused by insulin resistance leads to an initial compensatory hyperinsulinaemia, which maintains normoglycaemia until worsening β-cell failure gives rise to IGT or diabetes. Glucose tolerance returns to normal with effective lowering of growth hormone levels.

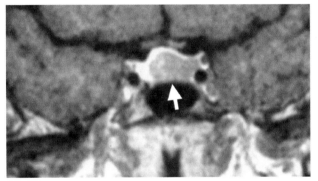

FIGURE 8.19
Large pituitary adenoma demonstrated by magnetic resonance imaging.

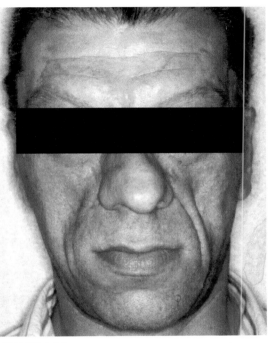

FIGURE 8.20
Acromegaly in a patient found to have a random blood glucose level of 13 mmol/L (234 mg/dL). Note the characteristic facies.

Phaeochromocytomas are tumours that arise from the chromaffin cells of the sympathetic nervous system, usually in the adrenal medulla. They secrete catecholamines, epinephrine (adrenaline) and norepinephrine (noradrenaline), and sometimes dopamine. Typically, hypertension, headaches, tachycardia and sweating occur. Up to 75% of patients have IGT or mild type 2-like diabetes that does not require insulin. Catecholamines have several anti-insulin effects, including inhibiting insulin secretion, stimulating glucagon secretion, stimulating liver and muscle glycogenolysis and adipose tissue lipolysis, and causing postreceptor resistance to insulin-stimulated glucose uptake.

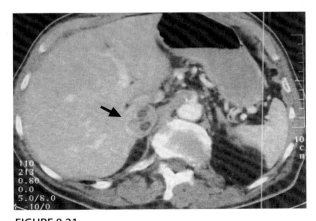

FIGURE 8.21
Phaeochromocytoma in a 75-year-old man demonstrated by computer tomography. The patient was admitted with chest pain, hypertension and a blood glucose level of 27 mmol/L (486 mg/dL).

HANDBOOK OF DIABETES 3RD EDITION

Glucagonomas are rare tumours of the islet α cells. They grow slowly, but are usually malignant. The most striking clinical features are weight loss and a characteristic rash, termed 'necrolytic migratory erythema'. There is also a tendency to thrombosis (pulmonary embolism is a common cause of death) and neuropsychiatric disturbances. Diabetes is caused by the enhanced gluconeogenesis and glycogenolysis induced by high glucagon concentrations.

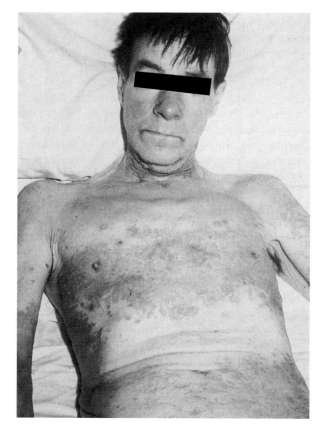

FIGURE 8.22
A patient with glucagonoma, showing characteristic necrolytic migratory erythema. Non-ketotic diabetes was controlled with low doses of insulin.

DIABETES CONTROL AND ITS MEASUREMENT

'Diabetic control' defines the extent to which metabolism in the diabetic patient differs from that in the non-diabetic person. Measurement traditionally has focused on blood glucose: 'good' glucose control refers to the maintenance of near-normal blood glucose concentrations throughout the day. However, many other metabolites are disordered in diabetes, and some, such as ketone bodies, are clinically useful. Metabolic control can be assessed in many ways: in addition to blood and urine glucose concentrations, measures of long-term control over the preceding weeks include glycated haemoglobin or fructosamine, while other indices of insulin deficiency include blood and urinary ketones.

Index	Main clinical use
Urine glucose	Only crude index of BG, 'last resort' in type 2 diabetes
Blood glucose • fasting • diurnal/circadian profiles	• Correlated with mean daily BG and HbA_{1c} in type 2 diabetes • Self-monitoring of BG, hospital assessment
Glycated haemoglobin	Glycaemic control (mean) over preceding 1–3 months
Glycated serum protein e.g. 'fructosamine'	Glycaemic control (mean) over preceding 2 weeks
Urine ketones	Insulin deficiency, warning of DKA
Other blood metabolites/hormones • cholesterol • triglyceride	• Cardiovascular risk factor • Cardiovascular risk factor

FIGURE 9.1
Some indices of diabetic control. BG, blood glucose; DKA, diabetic ketoacidosis.

Single blood glucose measurements are of little use in type 1 diabetes because of unpredictable variations in blood glucose throughout the day and from day to day. Serial, timed blood glucose samples are needed. In type 2 diabetes, however, blood glucose levels are elevated but not widely varying and reasonably consistent from day to day. A fasting or random blood glucose level in type 2 diabetes therefore relates reasonably closely to the mean blood glucose concentration and to glycated haemoglobin percentage (a measure of long-term control, see below).

FIGURE 9.2
Variations in plasma glucose concentrations over 2 days in a non-diabetic person, a type 1 diabetic patient (wide swings in glucose levels with little day-to-day consistency) and type 2 diabetes patient (similar profile to non-diabetic subject, but at a higher level and with greater postprandial peaks; fairly consistent from day to day).

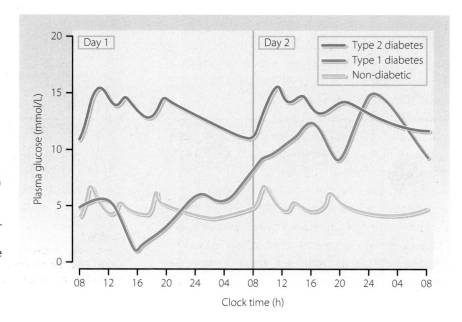

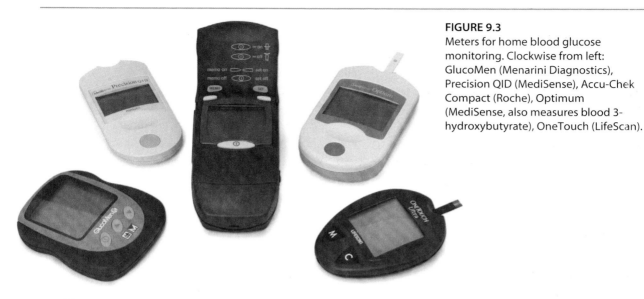

FIGURE 9.3
Meters for home blood glucose monitoring. Clockwise from left: GlucoMen (Menarini Diagnostics), Precision QID (MediSense), Accu-Chek Compact (Roche), Optimum (MediSense, also measures blood 3-hydroxybutyrate), OneTouch (LifeScan).

Self-monitoring of capillary blood glucose concentrations by patients at home, using enzyme-impregnated dry-reagent strips, is now an integral part of modern diabetes management, especially for those who receive insulin injections. Strips usually contain glucose oxidase and peroxidase, together with a chromogen that changes colour in proportion to the glucose concentration. The colour can be assessed visually, by comparison with a printed chart or measured in a reflectance meter. Newer, electrochemically based strips generate a current rather than a colour change. Such meters are particularly useful for patients with colour vision defects because of retinopathy or other causes.

Several devices that contain a spring-loaded lancet are available for obtaining a blood sample. The fingers are the usual sites of sampling, the sides being less sensitive than the pulp. Training and correct technique are important for reliable results. A major reason for poor patient compliance and a low frequency of testing is the discomfort of testing the fingers, and in recent years devices have become available that operate with a much smaller blood volume and offer the option of testing at alternative sites that are much less densely innervated than the fingers – forearm and upper arm, abdomen, calf and thigh. However, there can be discrepancies in the values measured at the finger and alternative sites when the blood glucose is changing rapidly (e.g. the forearm value sometimes being delayed compared to the finger).

FIGURE 9.4
Automatic lancet devices for obtaining capillary blood samples. From left: Accu-Chek Soft Clix (Roche), OneTouch UltraSoft (LifeScan), AutoLancet (MediSense).

Glycosuria occurs when blood glucose levels exceed the renal threshold for glucose, approximately 10 mmol/L (180 mg/dL). However, urine glucose testing is an unreliable way to assess blood glucose control because the renal threshold varies between and within patients, fluid intake affects urine glucose concentrations and the result does not reflect the blood glucose at the time of testing, but over the time that urine has accumulated in the bladder. A negative urine test cannot distinguish between hypoglycaemia, normoglycaemia and moderate hyperglycaemia.

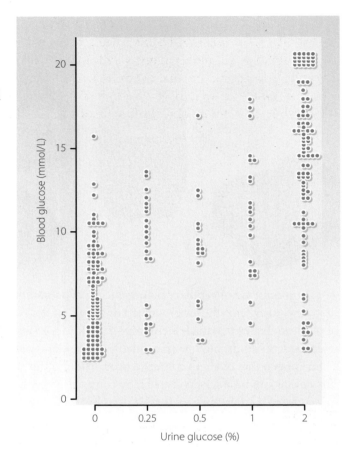

FIGURE 9.5
Blood glucose concentrations corresponding to various urine glucose tests (0–2%) in diabetic children.

Urine glucose testing still remains a reasonable option in stable type 2 diabetic subjects treated by diet or oral agents, particularly in those unable or unwilling to perform blood glucose tests. However, it should be supplemented by regular blood glucose and glycated haemoglobin tests in the clinic or doctor's office.

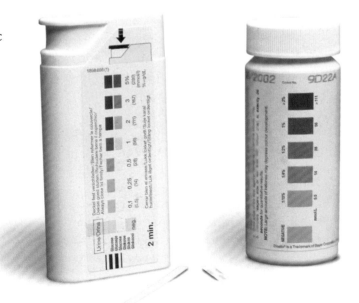

FIGURE 9.6
Urine testing strips.

Glycated haemoglobin (GHb) percentage is a measure of integrated glycaemic control over the preceding 2–3 months, and especially the last month. A number of adducts are formed by the slow, non-enzymatic attachment of sugars to adult haemoglobin (HbA); HbA_{1c} is present in the largest amount (60–80%) and is the result of attachment of glucose to the N terminal of the β chain of haemoglobin.

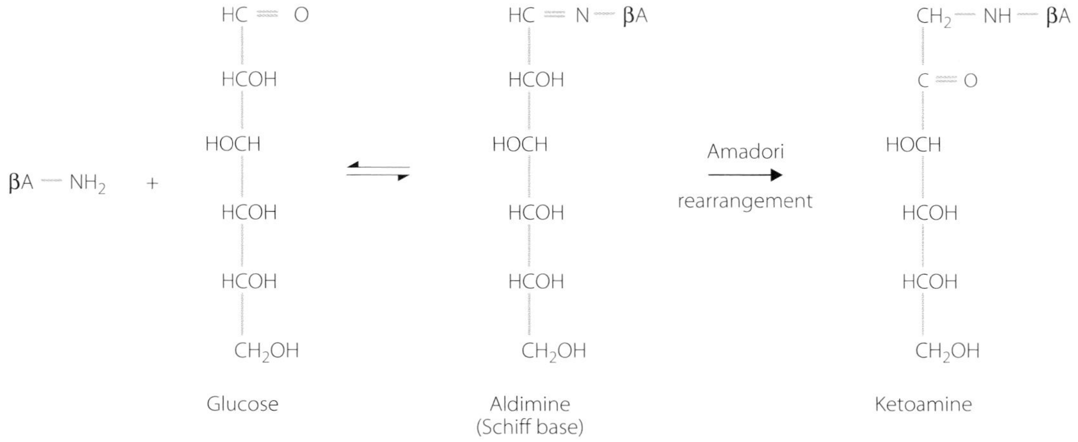

FIGURE 9.7
The formation of glycated haemoglobin (HbA_{1c}). Glucose forms a Schiff base linkage to the N-terminal valine of the β-chain of haemoglobin, which rearranges to yield the stable ketoamine product.

G Hb can be measured by several methods in the laboratory, including high-performance anion-exchange liquid chromatography (HPLC), gel electrophoresis, affinity chromatography (based on the interaction of the *cis*-diol of the sugar moiety of GHb with an immobilized boronic acid derivative) and immunoassay. The reference range in the non-diabetic population is about 4.5–6.5%, but normal ranges have not been interchangeable between laboratories because of assay variations and the difficulty of standardization. Whichever GHb species is measured, values are now usually reported as 'HbA$_{1c}$ equivalents', aligned to the HbA$_{1c}$ method used in the Diabetes Control and Complications Trial (DCCT, see Chapter 14); these are more reliably comparable between different laboratories.

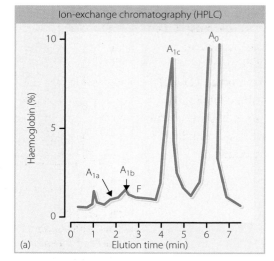

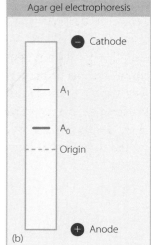

FIGURE 9.8
Methods for determination of glycated haemoglobin analysis. (a) Ion-exchange chromatography, (b) agar gel electrophoresis, (c) affinity chromatography and (d) immunoassay (latex agglutination inhibition).

In clinical practice, HbA$_{1c}$ provides an objective measure of long-term glycaemic control in a single measurement. It confirms to the physician the patterns in control seen with the patient's home blood glucose results, and reveals inconsistencies between self-monitored values and the patient's clinical history and hospital or office glucose results. As a result of the links established between control and tissue complications by major trials in type 1 (DCCT, see Chapter 14) and type 2 diabetes (UK Prospective Diabetes Study, see Chapter 14), the HbA$_{1c}$ level can also be regarded as a risk factor for development of microangiopathy.

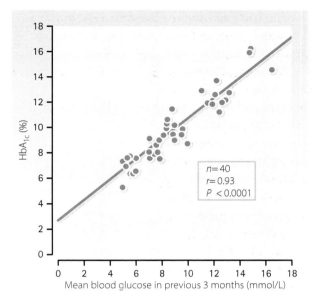

FIGURE 9.9
Correlation in type 1 diabetic patients between blood glucose concentration over the preceding 3 months and glycated haemoglobin (HbA$_{1c}$) level.

The American Diabetes Association recommends that the goal of diabetes therapy should be to achieve an HbA$_{1c}$ <7%, and that treatment action should be taken when values are consistently >8%. In the DCCT, the mean plasma glucose concentration could be related to HbA$_{1c}$ in a way that aids understanding of the clinical meaning of HbA$_{1c}$ as an index of overall glycaemia.

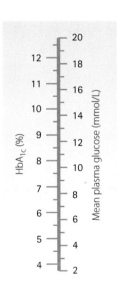

FIGURE 9.10
The correspondence between HbA$_{1c}$ and mean plasma glucose concentration in the Diabetes Control and Complications Trial (DCCT).

Serum fructosamine is a measure of glycated serum proteins, mostly albumin, and is an index of glycaemic control over the previous 2–3 weeks, the lifetime of albumin. Colorimetric assays for fructosamine, which are usually adaptable for automated analysers, are based on glycated protein acting as a reducing agent in alkaline solution. The reference range for non-diabetic subjects is about 205–285 μmol/L. Fructosamine generally correlates well with HbA$_{1c}$, except when the control has changed recently. It is useful when control is changing rapidly (e.g. in diabetic pregnancy). With recent improvements in HbA$_{1c}$ assays, which now are harmonized to a single standard method, fructosamine is used less frequently.

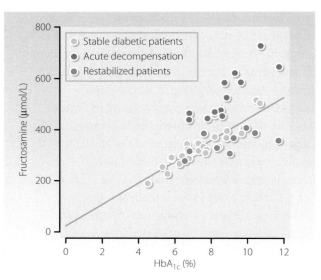

FIGURE 9.11
Correlation of serum fructosamine and HbA$_{1c}$ in diabetic patients. The correlation is best in stable diabetic patients and worst in those whose control has changed markedly in recent weeks.

Ketone measurements reflect severe insulin deficiency and warn against impending ketoacidosis. Most ketone tests are based on nitroprusside (Rothera's test), which produces a purple colour with acetoacetate and acetone. The tests do not react with 3-hydroxybutyric acid – which is quantitatively the most important ketone body in diabetic ketoacidosis (DKA). Nitroprusside-based ketone tests are thus relatively insensitive at detecting DKA. Test strips and electrochemical meters that measure 3-hydroxybutyrate are now available, but are not yet commonly used. Urine ketone testing is useful during acute illness, pregnancy and when symptoms of DKA are present (abdominal pain, nausea and vomiting), but many healthy individuals also have detectable urinary ketones in the fasting state, and ketones can persist in the urine long after the resolution of DKA.

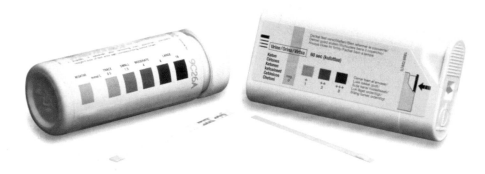

FIGURE 9.12
Urine ketone strips.

Glucose sensors for continuous *in vivo* monitoring of glycaemia in diabetic patients are now entering clinical practice. Minimally invasive sensors include needle-type enzyme electrodes that are implanted subcutaneously and measure interstitial glucose concentrations for up to 3 days. Data from the sensor are recorded by a portable monitor and later downloaded to a computer for analysis. Another technology uses a subcutaneously implanted microdialysis probe to sample interstitial fluid glucose levels. In reverse iontophoresis, a small current is passed between skin-surface electrodes and draws fluid to the surface for glucose assay. A watch-type device based on this technology has recently entered clinical practice.

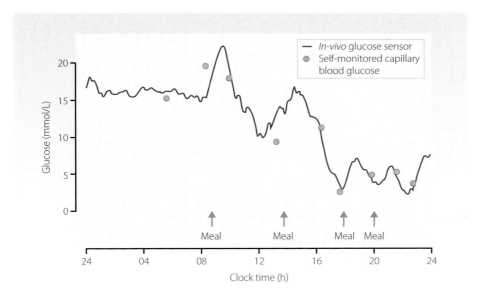

FIGURE 9.13
Continuous *in-vivo* glucose sensing in a type 1 diabetic subject with an implanted enzyme electrode (Medtronic MiniMed Continuous Glucose Monitoring System). Note episodes of postprandial hyperglycaemia, not detected by capillary blood glucose monitoring.

MANAGEMENT OF TYPE 1 DIABETES

Modern management of the type 1 diabetic patient, often called 'optimized' or 'intensive' therapy, encompasses a package of measures that includes 'physiological' insulin replacement (see below), assessment of glycaemic control by blood glucose self-monitoring and hospital and/or office tests, insulin dosage adjustments, a healthy diet and diabetes education.

Optimized or intensive insulin treatment

- Physiological insulin regimen
- Assessment of control
- Dosage adjustment
- Diet and exercise
- Diabetes education

FIGURE 10.1
Optimized or intensive insulin treatment.

The philosophy of insulin replacement is to mimic with exogenous insulin administration the insulin secretion pattern in the non-diabetic person – so-called 'physiological' insulin delivery. After eating, there is normally a rapid increase in plasma insulin, which limits postprandial glycaemia by stimulating peripheral glucose uptake. During the overnight fast and between meals, low steady levels of insulin (often called the 'basal' supply) are sufficient to restrain hepatic glucose output and maintain normoglycaemia.

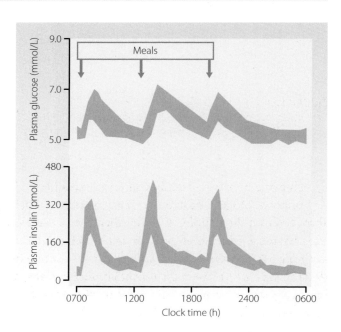

FIGURE 10.2
Normal plasma glucose and insulin profiles. Shaded areas represent mean ±2 SD.

Insulin is usually injected subcutaneously and regimens employ short-acting (unmodified, 'soluble' or 'regular') insulin, or a rapid-acting insulin analogue, to simulate normal mealtime insulin levels, while delayed-acting insulin is used to provide the background or basal concentration. This is sometimes called the 'basal-bolus' strategy.

FIGURE 10.3
Basal-bolus insulin regimen.

HANDBOOK OF DIABETES *3RD EDITION*

Until the 1980s, insulin was extracted and purified from the pancreas of cattle and pigs. Animal insulins are still in use, but have been superseded for the majority of patients in many countries by human-sequence insulin. Human insulin is manufactured by recombinant DNA technology (i.e. by inserting into *Escherichia coli* bacteria or yeast cells either synthetic genes for the insulin A chain and B chain, or the proinsulin gene or a proinsulin-like precursor). Fermentation results in large amounts of the recombinant protein, which can be converted into insulin and purified.

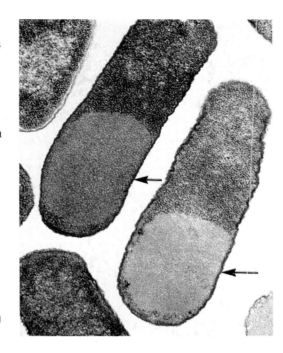

FIGURE 10.4
Transmission electron micrograph of *Escherichia coli* cells showing accumulation of expressed insulin precursor protein (arrows).

Achieving normoglycaemia with insulin injections is frustrated by several pharmacological problems. Firstly, subcutaneously injected insulin is absorbed into the peripheral rather than the portal bloodstream; thus, effective insulinization of the liver can be achieved only at the expense of systemic hyperinsulinaemia. Moreover, short-acting insulins are absorbed too slowly to mimic precisely the normal prandial peaks, and must therefore be injected about 30 minutes before the meal so that the peak of blood insulin corresponds with the blood glucose rise after a meal.

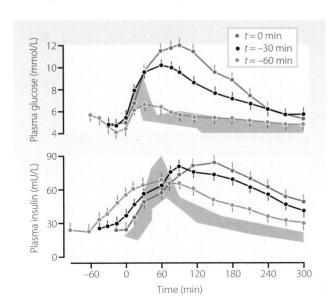

FIGURE 10.5
Soluble insulin should be injected 30 minutes before eating to optimize prandial glucose profiles. Glucose and insulin responses (mean ± SEM) are shown for eight type 1 diabetic patients given soluble insulin 0, 30 or 60 minutes before eating. The shaded areas represent mean ±2 SD in eight non-diabetic controls.

This slow absorption occurs because, on injection, native insulin remains in the self-associated hexameric form, which is too large to be absorbed into the circulation. Time is needed for diffusion and dilution to allow dissociation of the hexamer into dimers and monomers that can be absorbed readily.

FIGURE 10.6
Putative events in the subcutaneous tissue after subcutaneous injection of regular human insulin.

'Monomeric' insulin analogues have been introduced in recent years to speed the absorption of subcutaneously injected insulin. Using genetic and protein engineering techniques, changes are made in the amino-acid sequence of insulin that reduce the tendency to self-associate. The first monomeric insulin to be marketed was lispro (Humalog®; Eli Lilly), in which the B28 lysine and B29 proline residues of native insulin are reversed (B28 Lys, B29 Pro insulin). Another analogue, aspart (NovoRapid®; Novo Nordisk), has the structure B28 Asp, B29 Lys insulin. Rapid-acting insulin analogues have a peak action about 1–2 hours after injection and can be injected at the start of the meal. The duration of action is shorter than for regular insulin and this reduces the risk of late postprandial hypoglycaemia.

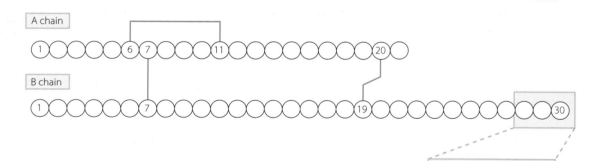

FIGURE 10.7
Structures of the rapid-acting insulin analogues, lispro and aspart, compared with native human insulin.

Intermediate- or delayed-acting insulins are of three main types. Isophane is an insoluble suspension of insulin made by combining insulin with the highly basic protein protamine, together with zinc ions, at neutral pH. It is also called NPH (neutral protamine Hagedorn, after the Hagedorn Laboratories in Copenhagen, where it was developed in the 1940s). Lente insulins are insoluble insulin suspensions made by adding excess zinc ions to insulin. Both isophane and lente have a duration of action of about 8–12 hours after subcutaneous injection. A variation of lente called ultralente, with larger, more insoluble crystals, has a duration of more than 24 hours when made from beef insulin, but its human formulation is similar in duration to that of isophane and lente insulins.

Longer-acting insulin analogues are being actively developed, and the first has been introduced into clinical service. Insulin glargine (Lantus®; Aventis) is made by substituting basic amino acids at the C-terminus of the B chain of insulin, thus altering the isoelectric point (where the protein is least soluble) from pH 5.4 to 7.4. At a slightly acidic pH in the vial, glargine is soluble, but after subcutaneous injection it precipitates as microcrystals at physiological pH. Detemir (NN304®; Novo Nordisk), another long-acting analogue undergoing clinical evaluation, is acylated with a fatty acid at the C terminus of the insulin B chain. The fatty acid binds to albumin, which slows insulin absorption and prolongs the circulation time.

Insulin class	Time of action (h)			Species or origin
	Onset	Peak	Duration	
Short-acting insulins				
• Monomeric (lispro, aspart)	<0.5	0.5–2.5	3.0–4.5	Synthetic
• Short-acting (soluble, regular)	0.2–0.5	1.0–3.0	4.0–8.0	Human, porcine, bovine
Intermediate-acting (delayed-action) insulins				
• Isophane (NPH)	1.0–2.0	4.0–6.0	8.0–12.0	Human, porcine, bovine
• Lente	1.0–2.0	4.0–8.0	8.0–14	Human, porcine, bovine
	1.0–3.0	5.0–10	10–24	Porcine, bovine
Long-acting insulins				
Ultralente	2.0–3.0	4.0–8.0	8.0–14	Human
	2.0–4.0	6.0–12	12–28	Bovine
Analogues (e.g. glargine)	0.75–1.5	Peakless	16-724	Synthetic

FIGURE 10.8 Duration of action of insulins.

The time–action profile of glargine does not show the pronounced peak found with isophane and lente insulins and has a duration of action >24 hours. It is usually injected once daily, at the same time each day, and has been shown to cause less nocturnal hypoglycaemia and less variable fasting blood glucose concentrations than isophane insulin.

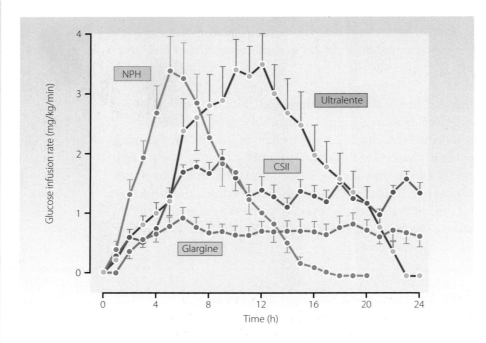

FIGURE 10.9
Action profiles of neutral protamine Hagedorn (NPH), ultralente, glargine and continuous subcutaneous insulin infusion (CSII).

A variety of premixed or 'biphasic' insulins are available, in which fixed ratios of short-acting and isophane insulin have been mixed in the vial by the manufacturer. The 30% short-acting/70% isophane and 25/75 mixtures are the most popular. Regular and lente insulins cannot be mixed because the excess zinc transforms some of the regular insulin into a long-acting type. Mixtures of rapid-acting analogues and their protamine-retarded counterparts have also been introduced.

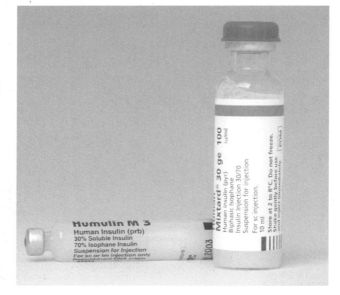

FIGURE 10.10
Premixed insulins.

The recommended sites for insulin injection are the subcutaneous tissue of the lower abdomen, upper outer thighs, upper outer arms and the buttocks. Disposable plastic syringes with a fine needle can be re-used for several injections, until the needle becomes blunt. Injection should be given into a pinched-up skin fold, penetrating no more than 3–5 mm to avoid inadvertent intramuscular administration (which accelerates absorption).

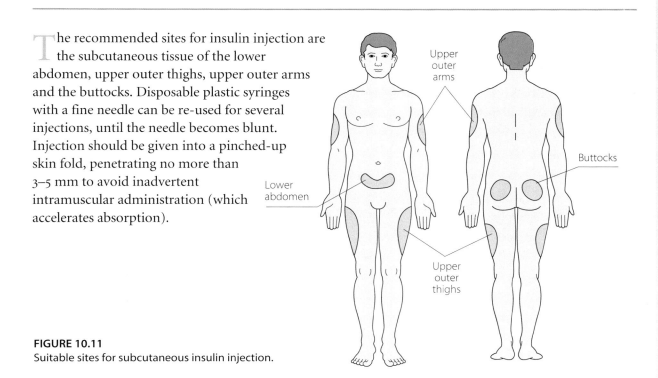

Upper outer arms

Buttocks

Lower abdomen

Upper outer thighs

FIGURE 10.11
Suitable sites for subcutaneous insulin injection.

Insulin absorption is fastest in the abdomen and slowest in the thigh and buttocks, and can be accelerated by exercise or taking a sauna. Short-acting insulin is best given into the abdomen (which is less susceptible to acceleration of absorption with exercise) and long-acting insulin into the thigh.

Repeated injection into the same subcutaneous site may, in the long term, give rise to an accumulation of fat (lipohypertrophy) because of the local trophic action of insulin. Lipohypertrophy can be unsightly and also increases the variability of insulin absorption; to avoid this, the site of insulin injection should be rotated within a given anatomical area. The affected lipohypertrophic area becomes painless to injection, thus being favoured by the patient and making the problem worse.

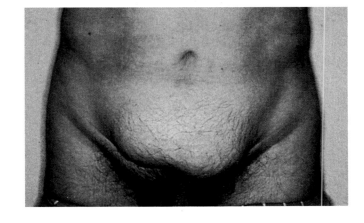

FIGURE 10.12
Lipohypertrophy at a habitually used insulin injection site.

HANDBOOK OF DIABETES 3RD EDITION

Another local reaction is lipoatrophy. This unsightly hollowing of the subcutaneous fat is thought to result from local deposition of insulin IgG immune complexes. With modern, highly purified insulins, which do not induce a significant immune response, lipoatrophy is hardly ever seen.

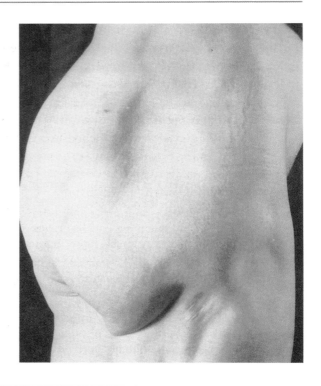

FIGURE 10.13
Extensive lipoatrophy in a 39-year-old woman treated over 20 years with various 'impure' insulin preparations.

Insulin 'pens' have become a popular option for injection therapy in recent years. The insulin is contained in a reservoir in the pen-shaped barrel, which also incorporates a fine needle. The main advantages of insulin pens include convenience and ease of injection, less painful injection (because the needle remains sharp for longer, as it is not reinserted through the rubber diaphragm of the insulin vial) and good patient acceptance – thereby encouraging multiple injection regimens.

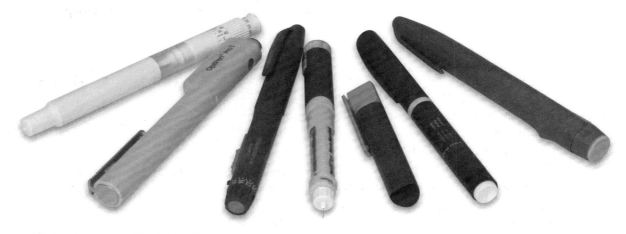

FIGURE 10.14
Insulin pens.

HANDBOOK OF DIABETES 3RD EDITION

Apopular insulin regimen for type 1 diabetic patients involves either short-acting regular insulin or a rapid-acting analogue given with each meal (or just with breakfast and the evening meal if lunch is small). Dosages are varied, generally according to the carbohydrate content of the meal, and adjusted by the postprandial blood glucose value. Isophane or lente are usually given twice daily. If the intermediate-acting insulin is injected with the evening meal, the peak insulin action at about 0100 hours tends to cause nocturnal hypoglycaemia at about 0100–0300 hours. Insulin sensitivity decreases in the few hours before breakfast because of surges of growth hormone during sleep. The effect of this, together with the waning of the previous evening's insulin, leads to fasting hyperglycaemia (the 'dawn phenomenon'). This problem can be countered by moving the delayed-action insulin injection to bedtime. Glargine, with its 24-hour action, is usually injected once daily; in some patients, its duration appears substantially shorter, and these cases benefit from twice-daily administration of glargine.

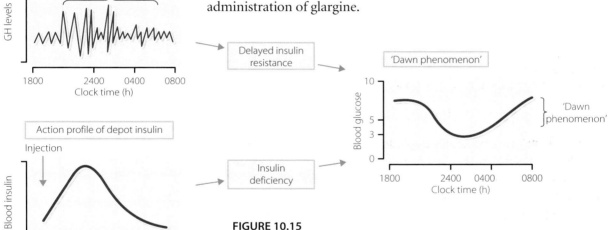

FIGURE 10.15
The 'dawn phenomenon'. A prebreakfast rise in blood glucose levels occurs because the growth hormone (GH) surges during sleep induce delayed insulin resistance. This effect can be accentuated if insulin levels run out overnight (e.g. from intermediate-acting insulin injected in the early evening).

Intensive therapy is appropriate in most type 1 diabetic patients, aiming for blood glucose levels of about 6.5–7.5 mmol/L (117–135 mg/dL) before meals and overnight, and of <9 mmol/L (162 mg/dL) 2 hours after main meals. Non-intensive therapy with somewhat higher target blood glucose levels may be suitable for very young or elderly patients, or those with disabling hypoglycaemia or other serious disease.

Time-points	Intensive	Non-intensive
Fasting Pre-meal Bedtime 03.00 hours	6.5–7.5 mmol/L	8.0–11.0 mmol/L
2 h after meal	< 9.0 mmol/L	Not needed
HbA₁c	6.5–7.0%	8.0–9.0%

FIGURE 10.16
Blood glucose targets in intensive and non-intensive insulin treatment schedules.

Alternative insulin delivery systems

Artificial insulin delivery systems can be either 'open-loop', in which insulin infusion rates are preselected by the doctor or patient, or 'closed-loop', in which there is continuous glucose sensing and computer-regulated feedback control of insulin delivery (the so-called 'artificial pancreas'). Continuous subcutaneous insulin infusion (CSII) is an open-loop insulin delivery system in which a portable pump is used to infuse insulin subcutaneously at variable rates and thereby mimic non-diabetic insulin secretion – a basal rate throughout the 24 hours and patient-activated boosts at mealtimes. This achieves excellent metabolic control. The basal rate can be changed at preset times, most usefully an increase during the night to counter the dawn phenomenon.

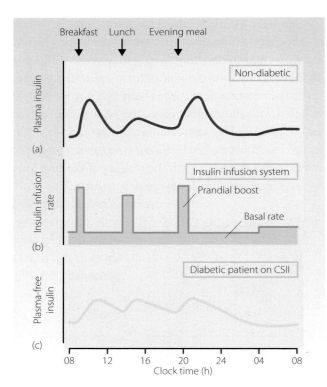

FIGURE 10.17
The aim with open-loop insulin delivery systems is to mimic non-diabetic insulin secretion (a), by infusing insulin at variable basal rates throughout the 24 hours, with patient-activated boosts at meals (b). (c) The plasma free insulin concentrations in a patient treated by continuous subcutaneous insulin infusion (CSII).

Battery-driven syringe pumps deliver insulin via a fine plastic cannula, which terminates in a subcutaneously implanted needle or flexible catheter. The pump is usually worn around the waist with the infusion cannula sited in the abdomen. Monomeric insulin (e.g. lispro or aspart) is now the pump insulin of choice.

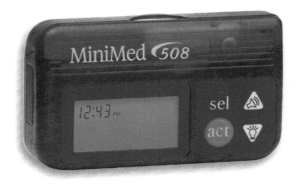

(a)

FIGURE 10.18
Insulin infusion pumps: (a) Medtronic MiniMed pump; (b) Disetronic pump.

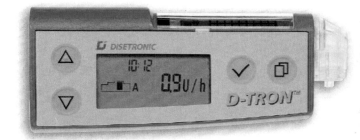

(b)

HANDBOOK OF DIABETES *3RD EDITION*

A typical strategy for starting pump therapy is to calculate the infusion rates by reducing the patient's usual total daily insulin dose on injection therapy by 20%, allocating one-half to the basal rate (about 0.9 U/h in adults, 13 mU/kg/h in children) and the other half divided between the three main meals. With monomeric insulin, boosts are given at the time of eating. Basal insulin rates can be adjusted by measuring blood glucose when fasting and at 0300 hours, and the prandial insulin by the blood glucose 90–120 minutes after a meal. Carbohydrate counting is valuable for adjusting the prandial boost to the size of the meal: generally, 1 U should be given per 15 g carbohydrate, with greater dosages with insulin resistance (e.g. adolescents, 1 U/10 g) and less for relatively insulin-sensitive subjects (e.g. small children, 1 U/20 g).

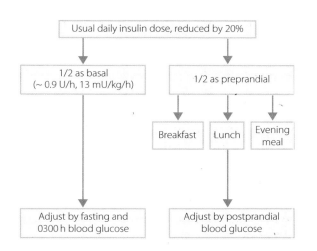

FIGURE 10.19
An infusion strategy for starting patients on continuous subcutaneous insulin infusion (CSII).

The best-established clinical indication for a trial of CSII is type 1 diabetic patients who have failed to achieve strict glycaemic control on multiple (intensive) insulin injection therapy because of frequent and unpredictable hypoglycaemia. CSII is extremely effective at reducing the frequency of serious hypoglycaemia in type 1 diabetes. A marked dawn phenomenon during optimized multiple injection therapy is also considered an indication by many physicians, though this can often be avoided with proper timing of bedtime isophane or the use of glargine.

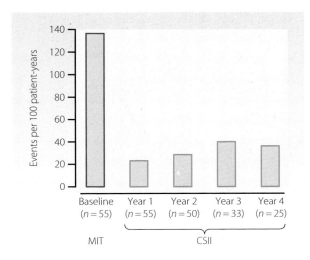

FIGURE 10.20
Frequency of severe hypoglycaemic events in 55 type 1 diabetic subjects treated by multiple-injection therapy (MIT) at baseline and then by continuous subcutaneous insulin infusion (CSII).

Prerequisites for CSII

Patients should be:

Willing

Motivated

Able to perform the procedures involved in CSII

Able to perform frequent blood glucose self-monitoring

Without significant psychological problems

Under the supervision of a health-care team experienced in CSII

Specific indications

Type 1 diabetic subjects who have failed to achieve good control with multiple-injection therapy (includes re-education, dietary advice, etc.), because of:

Frequent hypoglycaemia

A marked dawn phenomenon

All candidates for CSII should be motivated, compliant and willing to perform frequent blood glucose self-monitoring. A full education programme is necessary and CSII should be initiated and supervised by a health-care team that consists of a physician with a special interest in pump therapy, a specialist diabetes nurse and a dietitian. All must be experienced in the procedures of CSII.

FIGURE 10.21
The clinical indications for continuous subcutaneous insulin infusion (CSII).

Totally implantable pumps that deliver insulin into the peritoneal cavity or a central vein are still at an experimental stage. Overall glycaemic control (e.g. HbA$_{1c}$) tends to be similar to that during multiple insulin injection therapy or CSII, but with reduced fluctuations and fewer hypoglycaemic episodes. The routine use of implantable pumps has been limited by cost, the relative invasiveness of the procedure and some complications, such as catheter blockage by aggregated insulin. Recent improvements include specially formulated, more stable pump insulins, which are reducing complications. One of the few clinical indications is the management of rare cases of 'brittle' diabetes characterized by apparent resistance to subcutaneous insulin and often a normal sensitivity to intravenous insulin (a 'syndrome' that, in many cases, results from deliberate or inadvertent poor compliance with insulin treatment).

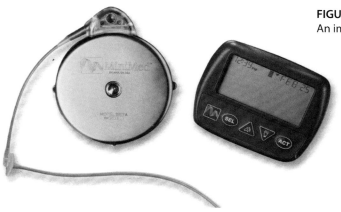

FIGURE 10.22
An implantable insulin pump (Medtronic MiniMed).

Trials are under way of insulin that can be inhaled as either an aerosolized dry powder or a liquid formulation, using mechanically or electronically controlled inhaler devices. Inhaled insulin is absorbed more quickly than regular subcutaneous insulin injections (peak activity about 30 minutes), but its bioavailability is only about 10–20%. It is thus suitable for mealtimes. Inhaled insulin is not yet available commercially.

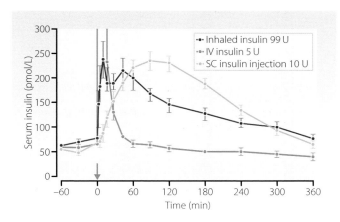

FIGURE 10.23

Serum insulin concentrations after the administration of insulin by inhalation, or by intravenous (IV) or subcutaneous (SC) injection of short-acting human insulin.

The starting points and mainstays of treatment for type 2 diabetes are diet and other modifications of lifestyle, such as increasing exercise and stopping smoking. The major aims are not only to reduce the weight of obese patients and improve glycaemic control, but also to reduce risk factors for cardiovascular disease (CVD), such as hyperlipidaemia and hypertension, which accounts for 70–80% of deaths in type 2 diabetes.

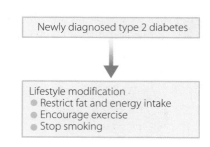

FIGURE 11.1 Management of type 2 diabetes: the initial measures.

Weight loss is achieved by decreasing total energy intake and/or increasing physical activity and thus energy expenditure. Gradual weight loss is preferred – not more than 0.5–1 kg/week. For effective weight loss and improvement in glycaemic control, the amount of energy restriction is more important than dietary composition, though compliance may be greater with high monounsaturated fat diets.

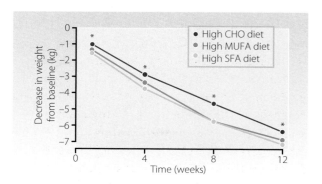

FIGURE 11.2
Change in weight during energy restriction is similar with high carbohydrate diet (CHO), high monounsaturated fatty acid (MUFA) diet and high saturated fatty acid (SFA) diet.

Anti-obesity drugs have so far played only a minor part in the management of the obese diabetic patient. *Sibutramine* is a centrally acting serotonin- and norepinephrine-reuptake inhibitor that acts as an appetite suppressant. It has contraindications (hypertension), potential drug interactions and requires careful monitoring, and little information on long-term efficacy and safety. *Orlistat* acts locally in the gastrointestinal tract, where it blocks enzymatic digestion of triglyceride by inhibiting pancreatic lipase. The absorption of up to 30% of ingested fat is thus prevented. Orlistat can induce significant weight loss in obese type 2 diabetic patients during a year's treatment, though weight may be regained subsequently. Gastrointestinal side-effects are common, including flatulence, steatorrhoea and, occasionally, faecal incontinence. A diet rich in fruit and vegetables is needed to avoid fat-soluble vitamin deficiency. Orlistat should be started only if diet alone has produced ≥2.5 kg weight loss over 1 month and should be discontinued if weight loss is <5% after 12 weeks.

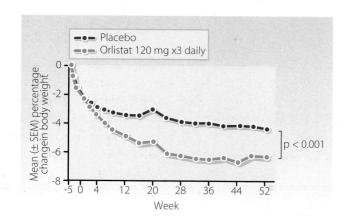

FIGURE 11.3
Effect of Orlistat in type 2 diabetic patients.

The dietary recommendations are essentially the same for type 1 and type 2 diabetes – and, indeed, follow a healthy eating plan suitable for the entire population. Saturated fat should be reduced and replaced with monounsaturated fat such as olive oil or polyunsaturated fats. n-6 polyunsaturated fat, found in vegetable oils, is also beneficial for lowering cholesterol and improving glycaemic control. Dietary cholesterol may be especially detrimental in the diabetic population, so the consumption of foods such as eggs should be limited. Fish oils are rich in n-3 fatty acids and have lower triglyceride levels, and there is evidence that higher fish intake is associated with less CVD in diabetes; accordingly, 2–3 servings of fish per week are recommended. Simple dietary guidelines in the form of recommended foods are normally best for patients, and are better understood than measures of fat, carbohydrate or protein. 'Diabetic' foods that contain sorbitol or fructose as sweetener are not recommended. Sucrose need not be banned from the diabetic diet, and a moderate amount for sweetening is acceptable. The focus of dietary plans should be on balancing energy intake to energy expenditure and the quality of fat and carbohydrate, rather than the quantity alone. Foods that normal improve glycaemic control and CVD risk are whole grains (brown rice, whole-wheat breads, oats) and high-fibre foods (grains, cereals, fruits, vegetables and nuts).

- Quench thirst with water or other sugar-free drinks
- Eat regular meals, avoiding fried and very sugary foods
- Eat plenty of vegetables
- Have high-fibre and low glycaemic index foods, including whole grains, legumes or brown rice as the main part of each meal
- Limit consumption of high glycaemic index starchy foods, such as mashed potatoes and white bread
- Eat plenty of whole fruit
- Limit consumption of animal products with high amounts of cholesterol and saturated fat, such as red meat, eggs, liver and high-fat dairy products, and substitute them with lean meat, fish, poultry (without skin) and low-fat dairy products
- For snacks between meals, avoid convenience foods such as biscuits, cake or confectionery (which are high in saturated and trans-fats and salt); use nuts and fruits for snacks instead
- Use natural liquid vegetable oils for cooking, baking and frying instead of vegetable shortenings (solid vegetable fat, high in saturates and trans-fatty acids)
- Use trans-fat-free or soft margarine instead of stick (hardened) margarine or butter
- Be aware of the portion size of a meal, especially when eating in a restaurant. Do not overeat
- If blood glucose control is satisfactory, light to moderate drinking of alcohol (1 unit per day for women and 1–2 for men) is fine, but drink alcoholic beverages with a meal

FIGURE 11.4
Practical food recommendations for diabetic patients.

In small quantities, alcohol has a protective effect on CVD, as it increases high-density lipoprotein cholesterol concentration, decreases coagulation factors and enhances insulin sensitivity. For those diabetic patients who choose to drink alcohol, light to moderate drinking with meals should not be discouraged, except in those with severe hypoglycaemia, hyperlipidaemia, hypertension, painful neuropathy, erectile dysfunction or pancreatic disease. Recommended alcohol intake is no more than 3 units/day in men and 2 units/day in women.

Cigarette smoking markedly enhances CVD risk in diabetes and should be discouraged vigorously. Stopping smoking is at least as effective in reducing CVD in diabetes as reducing cholesterol and controlling blood pressure and glycaemia.

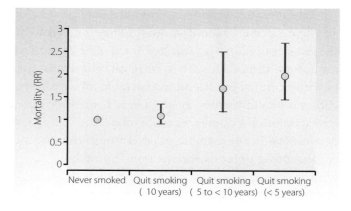

FIGURE 11.5
Relative risks (RRs) of total mortality by duration of smoking cessation among diabetic women.

Exercise should be tailored to the individual patient, according to physical condition and lifestyle, but simple advice might include moderate exercise as part of the daily schedule, such as walking for 30–60 minutes per day (preferably an extra 30–60 minutes). Exercise does not usually cause hypoglycaemia in type 2 diabetes (in contrast to type 1 diabetes), and therefore extra carbohydrate is generally unnecessary. Resistance exercise, such as weightlifting performed 2–3 times per week, may provide extra benefits over aerobic exercise; however, it should only be done with proper instruction, and progressively increased over some weeks, starting with a low-intensity workload. Regular exercise can reduce long-term mortality by 50–60% in type 2 diabetic people compared with patients with poor cardiorespiratory fitness.

There is a progressive decline in β-cell function and insulin sensitivity in type 2 diabetes, which results in deteriorating glycaemic control and the constant need to revise and intensify treatment. Diet and exercise are sufficient to achieve adequate glycaemic control in only about 10–20% of type 2 patients; when control worsens, an oral hypoglycaemic agent is generally introduced.

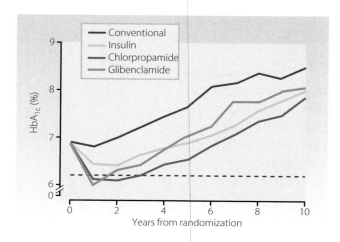

FIGURE 11.6
The progressive rise in median HbA$_{1c}$ with time in the 'conventionally treated' (diet) and 'intensively treated' (insulin, chlorpropamide and glibenclamide) groups in the United Kingdom Prospective Diabetes Study.

The particular drug treatment used in an individual patient with type 2 diabetes is determined by clinical judgement about the likely balance between β-cell impairment and insulin resistance in that particular case. Overweight and obese patients are likely to be insulin resistant: here, the insulin sensitizer metformin is a logical first choice. Thin patients generally have substantial β-cell failure, and sulphonylureas (which stimulate insulin secretion) are likely to be effective. β-cell function declines at about 4% per year, so sulphonylureas are less effective later in the disease. Additional oral agents have been introduced in recent years, including non-sulphonylurea secretagogues, thiazolidinedione insulin sensitizers and α-glucosidase inhibitors.

When oral agents are ineffective, insulin must be initiated to achieve satisfactory control. About 50% of type 2 diabetic patients need insulin within 6 years of diagnosis.

Action	Class	Drug	Mechanism
Increase insulin secretion	Sulphonylureas	Glibenclamide Gliclazide Glimepiride Glipizide Gliquidone Chlorpropamide Tolbutamide Tolazamide	Bind to sulphonylurea receptor on β cell, leading to closure of ATP-sensitive potassium channels
	Meglitinide analogues	Repaglinide Nateglinide	Bind to sulphonylurea receptor on β cell, leading to closure of ATP-sensitive potassium channels
Reduce insulin resistance	Thiazolidinediones	Pioglitazone Rosiglitazone	PPARγ agonist
Reduce insulin resistance, reduce hepatic glucose output	Biguanides	Metformin	Not known
Delay absorption of carbohydrate	α-Glucosidase inhibitors	Acarbose Guar gum	Inhibits α-glucosidase Increases fibre in diet
Reduce weight	Agents that reduce fat absorption	Orlistat	Inhibits pancreatic lipase
	Centrally acting agents	Sibutramine	Serotonin and norepinephrine reuptake inhibitor

FIGURE 11.7
Oral agents used in the treatment of type 2 diabetes.

Metformin is a derivative of guanidine, the active ingredient of goat's rue (*Galega officianalis*) – used as a treatment for diabetes in medieval Europe. Metformin increases insulin action (the exact mechanism is unclear), lowering glucose mainly by decreasing hepatic gluconeogenesis and thus glucose output. Unlike sulphonylureas, it does not cause hypoglycaemia or weight gain and, indeed, has some appetite-suppressing activity that may encourage weight loss. A typical starting dose of metformin is 500 mg daily or twice daily, rising to 850 mg thrice daily. Major side-effects are nausea, anorexia or diarrhoea, which affect about one-third of patients. Lactic acidosis is a rare, but serious, side-effect that carries high mortality. It can be avoided by not giving metformin to patients with renal, hepatic, cardiac or respiratory failure or those with a history of alcohol abuse.

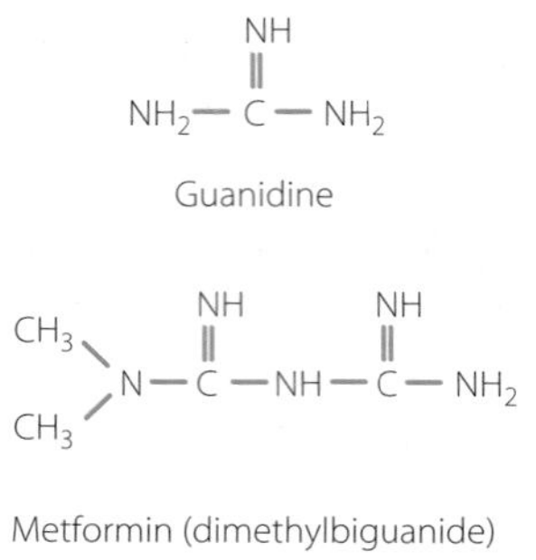

FIGURE 11.8
The chemical structures of guanidine and metformin.

Sulphonylureas stimulate insulin secretion by binding to sulphonylurea (SUR-1) receptors on the β-cell plasma membrane, which leads to closure of the ATP-sensitive K^+ channel (Kir6.2), membrane depolarization, opening of calcium channels, calcium influx and exocytosis of insulin granules. The most serious side-effect is hypoglycaemia, most likely with glibenclamide and long-acting preparations used in the elderly, particularly when there are additional risk factors such as excess alcohol intake, impaired renal function and intake of drugs that displace sulphonylureas from their plasma protein binding sites (salicylates, sulphonamides and monoamine oxidase inhibitors). Weight gain may also accompany sulphonylurea use.

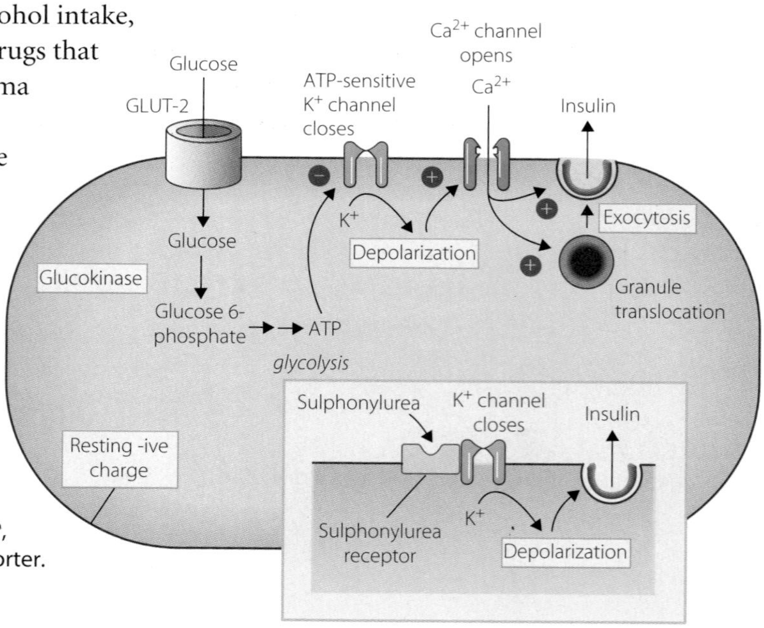

FIGURE 11.9
Mechanism by which glucose and sulphonylureas stimulate insulin secretion. ATP, adenosine triphosphate; GLUT, glucose transporter.

The so-called 'second generation' sulphonylureas, such as glipizide, gliclazide, glibenclamide (glyburide) and gliquidone, are most in use. These have a shorter half-life than the first sulphonylureas available (e.g. chlorpropamide) and have generally been given twice daily. This practice may need to be re-evaluated, since the effects depend on receptor binding of the drugs, which lasts longer than their plasma phase. Newer sulphonylureas include glimepiride, a once-daily preparation that may have an 'extrapancreatic', insulin-sparing action and a lower risk of hypoglycaemia.

Drug	Dose	Metabolism	Half-life	Comments
Chlorpropamide	125–500 mg	Hepatic ~ 20% excreted unchanged in urine	> 16 h	? Adverse effects on blood pressure Used successfully in the UKPDS
Tolbutamide	0.5–2 g	Hepatic < 20% excreted unchanged in urine	≈ 4 h	Concerns raised over possible increase in cardiovascular risk in UDPG trial
Glibenclamide (glyburide)	2.5–15 mg	Hepatic (~ 100%) Metabolites excreted in bile (50%) and urine (50%)	≈ 2 h	Risk of hypoglycaemia early in treatment Used successfully in the UKPDS
Gliclazide	40–320 mg	Hepatic < 5% excreted unchanged in urine	10–12 h	Useful first-line treatment Few long-term outcome data
Glipizide	2.5–40 mg	Hepatic (to inactive metabolites) < 10% excreted unchanged in urine	2–4 h	Sparse data on outcome
Glimepiride	1–6 mg	Hepatic: inactive metabolites excreted in urine (~ 60%) and faeces (~ 35%)	5–8 h	Sparse data on outcome
Gliquidone	30–180 mg	Hepatic (~ 100%), 95% excreted in bile and 5% in urine	1–4 h	Sparse data on outcome
Tolazamide	100–1000 mg	Active metabolites (with up to 70% activity of tolazamide) are excreted in urine	7 h	Sparse data on outcome

FIGURE 11.10
Sulphonylureas.

K_{ATP} channels are found in a variety of cells, with a common Kir6.2 unit, but different sulphonylurea receptors – SUR-1 in the β cell and SUR-2A in cardiac myocytes. These receptor types have different specificities towards different sulphonylureas. Gliclazide binds to the β-cell SUR isoform, but not to that in the cardiac myocyte. Glibenclamide binds to both the β cell and the cardiac SUR. The clinical significance of this is not clear, but there may be a potential for fewer extrapancreatic side-effects (including cardiac arrhythmias) with some sulphonylureas.

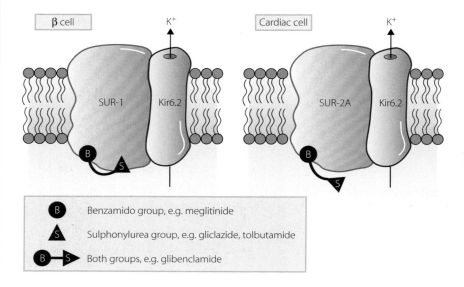

FIGURE 11.11
A model for sulphonylurea interaction with the ATP-sensitive K^+ channel on β cells and cardiac cells. The channel consists of two subunits: the K^+ pore (Kir6.2) to which ATP binds, and a regulatory subunit to which sulphonylureas bind [sulphonylurea receptor 1 (SUR-1) in the β cell and SUR-2A in the myocyte cell]. The β-cell receptor has two sites, one that accepts benzamido compounds and one that accepts the sulphonylurea group.

β cell K+ SUR-1 Kir6.2 B S

Cardiac cell K+ SUR-2A Kir6.2 B S

B	Benzamido group, e.g. meglitinide
S	Sulphonylurea group, e.g. gliclazide, tolbutamide
B → S	Both groups, e.g. glibenclamide

Meglitinides, such as repaglinide and nateglinide, are recently introduced non-sulphonylurea, short-acting agents that stimulate insulin secretion by binding to the benzamido site on the SUR (which is distinct from the site that binds classic sulphonylureas). They are used to control postprandial hyperglycaemia, and are taken before main meals. Nateglinide is not yet licensed as monotherapy, but can be used in combination with metformin (see below). In common with other insulin secretagogues, the meglitinides may cause hypoglycaemia.

Glibenclamide (Glyburide)

Meglitinides

Repaglinide

Nateglinide

FIGURE 11.12
Repaglinide and nateglinide are derived from the non-sulphonylurea benzamide portion of glibenclamide.

HANDBOOK OF DIABETES 3RD EDITION

The thiazolidinediones (TZD; also known as 'glitazones') were introduced into clinical practice in 1997. They are insulin sensitizers that enter the cell and bind to the peroxisome proliferator-activated receptor-γ (PPARγ), a nuclear receptor found predominantly in adipocytes, but also in muscle and liver. PPARγ forms a complex with the retinoid X receptor (RXR), and binding of a TZD leads to enhanced expression of certain insulin-sensitive genes, such as GLUT-4, lipoprotein lipase, fatty acid transporter protein and fatty acyl CoA synthase. This increases glucose uptake, increases adipocyte lipogenesis and decreases circulating fatty acid levels. There is also decreased production of the cytokine tumour necrosis factor α and of resistin, mediators that may be involved in the pathogenesis of insulin resistance (see Chapter 7).

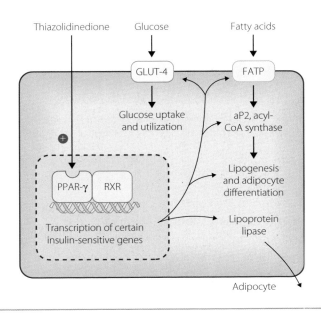

FIGURE 11.13
Mechanism of action of thiazolidinediones. These agents stimulate the peroxisome proliferator-activated receptor-γ (PPARγ) in the cell nucleus, mainly in the adipocyte. In conjunction with the retinoid X receptor (RXR), this promotes transcription of certain genes and increased expression of glucose transporter 4 (GLUT-4), fatty acid transporter protein (FATP), adipocyte fatty acid-binding protein (aP2), fatty acyl coenzyme A (CoA) synthase and other enzymes crucial in lipogenesis.

The first glitazone used, troglitazone, has been withdrawn because of an association with hepatotoxicity; subsequent thiazolidinediones (rosiglitazone and pioglitazone) do not cause this, but nonetheless regular liver function tests are recommended. They can be used as monotherapy (in the USA) or in combination with a sulphonylurea or metformin. Their use is associated with weight gain and fluid retention, and therefore they should not be given with insulin or to those with a history of cardiac failure or renal insufficiency.

Rosiglitazone

Pioglitazone

FIGURE 11.14
The chemical structures of the thiazolidinediones, rosiglitazone and pioglitazone.

α-Glucosidase inhibitors, such as acarbose (a complex oligosaccharide) and miglitol (a smaller saccharide), delay carbohydrate absorption by inhibiting disaccharidase enzymes in the gut and therefore lowering postprandial blood glucose concentrations. These agents have been limited by gastrointestinal side effects such as flatulence, diarrhoea and cramping, though these can diminish with time. Acarbose is only effective in those with adequate β-cell function and should therefore be used early in the course of type 2 diabetes. To be effective, it should be taken with the first mouthful of food.

FIGURE 11.15
Hydrolysis of starch, showing site of side-chain cleavage (α (1–6) glucosidase) that is inhibited by acarbose and miglitol)

It is common for many type 2 diabetic patients to progress from treatment by diet alone, to monotherapy with metformin or a sulphonylurea, then to a combination of the two (or the introduction of a 'glitazone'), before finally starting insulin. Insulin can be given alone or in combination with oral agents, almost always metformin. Several insulin regimens are suitable in type 2 diabetes; an initial basal regimen of isophane given once daily (e.g. at bedtime) or twice daily is popular, and twice-daily injections of premixed insulin (e.g. 30% short-acting/70% isophane) given with an insulin 'pen' are also convenient and effective in many patients. When obesity and insulin resistance predominate, the doses may range up to 2–3 units/kg.

Continuous subcutaneous insulin infusion (CSII, insulin pump therapy) has not yet been shown to be significantly more effective than multiple insulin injections in type 2 diabetes, though its use is being explored in some countries. Weight gain is a significant problem with insulin therapy in type 2 diabetes.

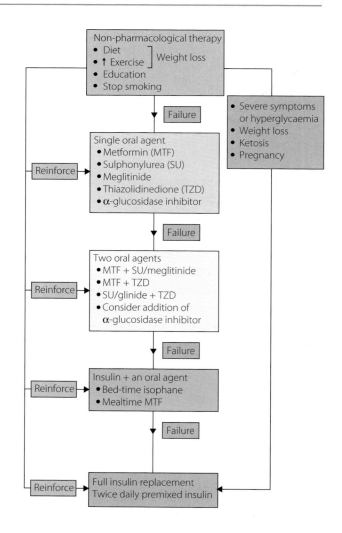

FIGURE 11.16
Algorithm for treating type 2 diabetes.

DIABETIC KETOACIDOSIS AND HYPEROSMOLAR NON-KETOTIC HYPERGLYCAEMIA

12

Diabetic ketoacidosis (DKA) is a state of severe uncontrolled diabetes caused by insulin deficiency, and requires emergency treatment with insulin and intravenous fluids. It is characterized by hyperglycaemia, hyperketonaemia and metabolic acidosis. DKA is a serious condition with a mortality estimated at 5–10% in Western countries, and particularly high in less specialized centres and in the elderly. Younger patients with type 1 diabetes are typically affected, but ketoacidosis can also be precipitated in patients with type 2 diabetes during severe infections and other illnesses.

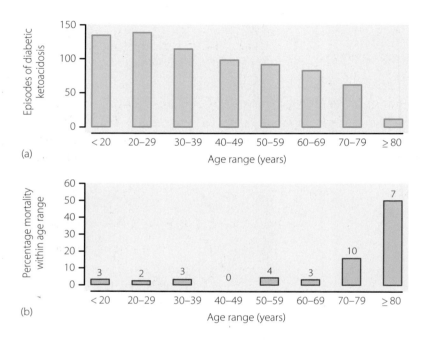

FIGURE 12.1
(a) Age distribution of 746 episodes of diabetic ketoacidosis (excluding paediatric cases). (b) Age distribution of deaths related to diabetic ketoacidosis ($n = 32$). Numbers of deaths in each age range are also shown.

DKA can also occur apparently spontaneously in some populations of African ancestry, who have an acute presentation typical of type 1 diabetes, but can then be controlled in the long term without insulin and have a clinical course that resembles type 2 diabetes. This is called 'ketosis-prone atypical diabetes mellitus'. The condition is well described in obese African–American adults and children, and has been termed 'Flatbush' diabetes, after the avenue in New York where the first patients lived. The immunogenetic markers of classic type 1 diabetes are absent.

FIGURE 12.2
Natural history and aetiology of ketosis-prone atypical diabetes.

Natural history

- Acute 'type 1-like' onset: severe hyperglycaemia and ketosis

- Subsequent 'type 2'-like course: declining insulin dosages

- Long-term 'remission' (50% of cases): well controlled by diet ± oral hypoglycaemic agents

- Relapses (ketosis, requiring temporary insulin treatment) may occur

Aetiology

- Impaired insulin secretion (partly reversible)

- Absence of type 1 diabetes immune markers (anti-GAD and islet-cell antibodies)

- Insulin resistance

GAD, glutamic acid decarboxylase.

Many factors can precipitate DKA in type 1 diabetes. Infections are commonly identified (about 30–40%), with new cases of diabetes accounting for about 10–20% (more so in children with diabetes – about 40%). Insulin errors and omissions and non-compliance are alarmingly common (about 15–30%). Frequently, there is no obvious cause.

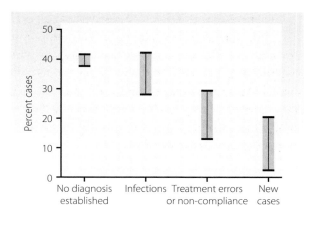

FIGURE 12.3
Precipitating causes of DKA, as reported in various studies.

Relative or absolute insulin deficiency in the presence of catabolic counter-regulatory stress hormones (particularly glucagon and catecholamines, but also growth hormone and cortisol) leads to hepatic overproduction of glucose and ketones. Lack of insulin combined with excess stress hormones promotes lipolysis, with the release of non-esterified fatty acids (NEFAs) from adipose tissue into the circulation. In the liver, fatty acids are partially oxidized to the ketone bodies acetoacetic acid and 3-hydroxbutyric acid, which contribute to the acidosis, and acetone (formed by the non-enzymatic decarboxylation of acetoacetate). The latter is volatile and often can be smelled on the breath of ketoacidotic patients.

Hyperglycaemia causes an osmotic diuresis that leads to dehydration and loss of electrolytes. Insulin deficiency further increases sodium depletion by decreasing renal sodium reabsorption. Metabolic acidosis leads to the exit of intracellular cellular potassium in exchange for hydrogen ions, and insulin deficiency also leads to potassium loss from cells and can raise plasma potassium levels.

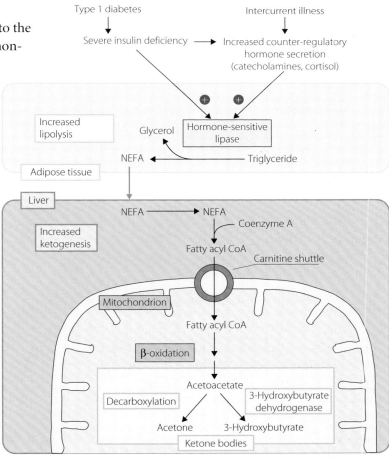

FIGURE 12.4
Mechanisms of ketoacidosis. NEFA, non-esterified fatty acids.

119

The symptoms of DKA include increasing polyuria and thirst, weight loss, weakness, drowsiness and eventually coma (in about 10% of cases). Abdominal pain can occur, particularly in the young. Physical signs include dehydration, hypotension, tachycardia and hypothermia. Acidosis stimulates the medullary respiratory centre, which causes deep and rapid (Kussmaul) respiration. The odour of acetone on the patient's breath (like nail-varnish remover) may be obvious to some, but many people are unable to detect it.

- Polyuria and nocturia; thirst
- Weight loss
- Weakness
- Blurred vision
- Acidotic (Kussmaul) respiration
- Abdominal pain, especially in children
- Leg cramps
- Nausea and vomiting
- Confusion and drowsiness
- Coma (10% of cases)

FIGURE 12.5
Clinical features of diabetic ketoacidosis.

The mechanism by which DKA induces coma is obscure, but impaired consciousness generally correlates with plasma glucose concentration and osmolarity; coma at presentation is associated with a worse prognosis. Coexisting causes of coma, such as stroke, head injury and drug overdose, should always be considered and excluded if appropriate. Cerebral oedema should be suspected when the conscious level declines during treatment (see below).

- Diabetic ketoacidosis
- Hyperosmolar non-ketotic hyperglycaemia
- Hypoglycaemia
- Lactic acidosis
- Other causes:

  Stroke (more common in diabetic patients)

  Post-ictal (including hypoglycaemia—convulsions also cause a self-correcting lactic acidosis)

  Cerebral trauma (may follow hypoglycaemia)

  Ethanol intoxication (may induce or exacerbate hypoglycaemia in diabetic patients).

  Drug overdose

FIGURE 12.6
Causes of coma or impaired consciousness in diabetic patients.

HANDBOOK OF DIABETES 3RD EDITION

D KA is a medical emergency. A rapid history, physical examination and bedside blood and urine tests should allow a tentative diagnosis in the emergency department and avoid treatment delays. Immediate bedside investigations should include blood glucose concentration and a test for the presence of urine or blood ketones with reagent strips, followed by laboratory measurements of blood glucose, urea, Na^+, K^+, Cl^-, bicarbonate (for calculation of the anion gap), arterial blood pH and gas tensions, and blood count, and blood and urine culture.

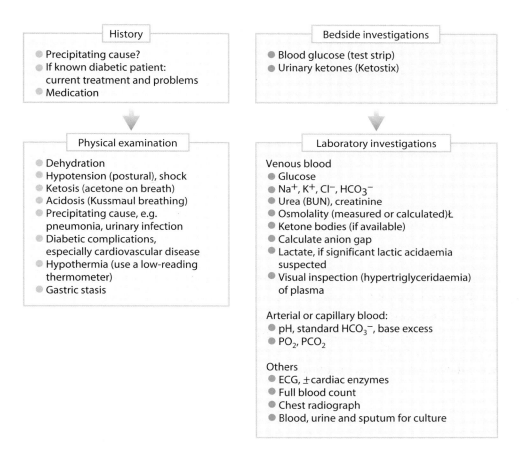

FIGURE 12.7
Flowchart for the investigation of diabetic ketoacidosis.

Treatment involves rehydration, initially with isotonic saline (with appropriate potassium supplements), switching to 5% dextrose when the blood glucose has fallen to ≤15 mmol/L (270 mg/dL). Short-acting insulin should be given ideally by low-dose intravenous infusion, initially 5–10 units/h until the blood glucose concentration falls to ≤15 mmol/L, then 1–4 units/h. Alternatively, insulin may be given by intramuscular injection (e.g. 5–10 units/h) until the blood glucose reaches ≤15 mmol/L. Potassium replacement is needed because insulin administration and the rising pH during initial treatment stimulate K^+ entry into the cells, which causes hypokalaemia and life-threatening arrhythmias and respiratory muscle weakness; generally, 20 mmol K^+ per litre of saline is given, adjusted by regular plasma K^+ measurements (see below). Intravenous bicarbonate, given in the hope of correcting acidosis, has not been proved to improve outcome and may predispose to cerebral oedema; it should be avoided.

Fluids and electrolytes

Volumes
- 1 L/h x 2–3, thereafter adjusted according to need

Fluids
- Isotonic ('normal') saline (150 mmol/L) generally
- Hypotonic ('half-normal') saline (75 mmol/L) if serum sodium exceeds 150 mmol/L (no more than 1–2 L—consider 5% dextrose with increased insulin if marked hypernatraemia)
- 5% dextrose 1 L 4–6-hourly when blood glucose has fallen to 15 mmol/L (severely dehydrated patients may require simultaneous saline infusion)
- Consider sodium bicarbonate (e.g. 700 mL of 1.26%, or 100 mL of 8.4% only if large vein cannulated), if pH < 7.0 (with extra potassium)

Potassium
- No potassium in first 1 L of fluid unless initial plasma potassium < 3.5 mmol/L
- Thereafter, add dosages below to each 1 L of fluid:
  If plasma K+:
  < 4.0 mmol/L, add 40 mmol KCl (severe hypokalaemia may require more aggressive KCl replacement)
  3.5–5.5 mmol/L, add 20 mmol KCl
  > 5.5 mmol/L, add no KCl

Insulin
Continuous intravenous infusion:
- 5–10 units/h (average 6 units/h) initially until blood glucose has fallen to ≤ 15 mmol/L. Thereafter, adjust rate (1–4 units/h usually) during dextrose infusion to maintain blood glucose 5–10 mmol/L until patient is eating again
- Intramuscular injections:
  20 units immediately, then 5–10 units/h until blood glucose has fallen to ≤ 15 mmol/L. Then change to 10 units 6-hourly subcutaneously until patient is eating again

Other measures
- Search for and treat precipitating cause (e.g. infection, myocardial infarction)
- Hypotension usually responds to adequate fluid replacement
- Central venous pressure monitoring in elderly patients or if cardiac disease present
- Pass nasogastric tube if conscious level impaired, to avoid aspiration of gastric contents
- Urinary catheter if conscious level impaired or no urine passed within 4 h of start of therapy
- Continuous ECG monitoring may warn of hyper- or hypokalaemia (potassium should be measured at 0, 2, and 6 h—and more often if indicated)
- Adult respiratory distress syndrome—mechanical ventilation (100% O_2, IPPV), avoid fluid overload
- Mannitol (up to 1 g/kg intravenously) if cerebral oedema suspected. Dexamethasone as alternative (induces insulin resistance). Consider cranial CT to exclude other pathology (e.g. cerebral haemorrhage, venous sinus thrombosis)
- Treat specific thromboembolic complications if they occur
- Meticulous clinical and biochemical record using a purpose-designed flow-chart

FIGURE 12.8
Guide to the initial treatment of diabetic ketoacidosis in adults.

HANDBOOK OF DIABETES 3RD EDITION

Complications of DKA include cerebral oedema, which occurs especially in children. It causes 'coning', in which swelling of the brain within the enclosed space of the cranium forces the base of the brain to herniate through the foramen magnum, leading to cardiorespiratory arrest. It is often fatal, and accounts for 50% of deaths in newly presenting DKA. The cellular mechanisms responsible for cerebral oedema in DKA are uncertain, but it tends to worsen after starting treatment with intravenous fluids and insulin, presenting clinically as a decline in conscious level, progressing to coma. The diagnosis should be confirmed by computed tomography or magnetic resonance scanning of the brain. A reasonable treatment approach includes slowing the rate of intravenous fluid infusion, avoiding hypotonic fluids, decreasing the insulin delivery rate and giving intravenous mannitol (0.2 g/kg over 30 minutes, repeated hourly if there is no improvement, or a single dose of 1 g/kg). Mechanical ventilation to remove carbon dioxide and improve acidosis has also been advocated.

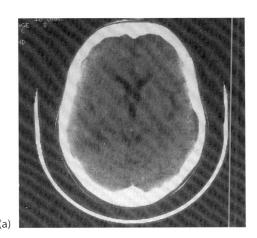
(a)

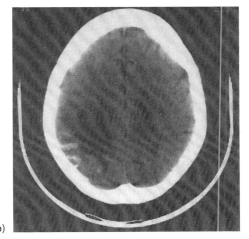
(b)

FIGURE 12.9
Brain computed tomograms of a 30-year-old woman who became comatose during treatment of diabetic ketoacidosis, showing both generalized cerebral oedema (a) and a parietal intracerebral haemorrhage (b). Cerebral oedema appears as loss of definition of normal brain texture, with compression of the ventricles and sulci.

Adult respiratory distress syndrome occasionally occurs in DKA, mostly in those under 50 years of age. The features include dyspnoea, tachypnoea, central cyanosis and arterial hypoxia. A chest radiograph shows bilateral infiltrates that resemble pulmonary oedema. Management involves intermittent positive-pressure ventilation and avoidance of fluid overload. Thromboembolism is a further potentially fatal complication of DKA, arising from dehydration, increased blood viscosity and coagulability. Prophylactic anticoagulation in DKA is not recommended, but established thromboembolism is treated conventionally.

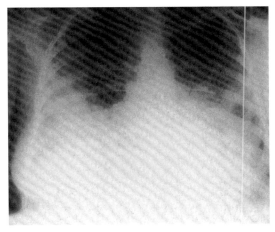

FIGURE 12.10
Adult respiratory distress syndrome. The chest radiograph shows typical bilateral shadowing, which resembles that of pulmonary oedema caused by left ventricular failure.

123

HANDBOOK OF DIABETES 3RD EDITION

Hyperosmolar non-ketotic hyperglycaemia (HONK) is characterized by the gradual development of marked hyperglycaemia [plasma glucose usually >35 mmol/L (630 mg/dL)], dehydration and prerenal uraemia, without significant ketosis and acidosis. It usually occurs in middle-aged or elderly patients with type 2 diabetes, about 25% of whom have previously undiagnosed diabetes. Certain ethnic groups (e.g. Afro-Caribbean) have a higher risk. The absence of ketones is incompletely explained, but may involve the suppression of lipolysis by hyperosmolarity, less pronounced counter-regulatory hormone responses in these patients, and the preservation of endogenous insulin secretion in type 2 diabetes. HONK is relatively uncommon, but carries a high mortality of about 15%, particularly in the elderly.

Hyperosmolar non-ketotic diabetic coma

- Marked hyperglycaemia
- Middle aged or elderly
- No ketosis or acidosis
- Often undiagnosed type 2 diabetes

FIGURE 12.11
Features of hyperosmolar non-ketotic diabetic coma.

Precipitating causes for HONK include infection, myocardial infarction and treatment with certain diabetogenic and/or dehydrating drugs, such as diuretics, β blockers and steroids. Other drugs associated with HONK are phenytoin, cimetidine, chlorpromazine and the anti-psychotic drugs clozapine and olanzapine. Omission of anti-diabetic drugs may also contribute. Thromboembolic complications are common, and rhabdomyolysis can occur. Treatment includes aggressive rehydration and electrolyte replacement, initially with isotonic (0.9%) saline (similar to the treatment of DKA), or 0.45% saline if the plasma sodium is >150 mmol/L. Insulin should be given by continuous intravenous infusion, initially at 6 units/h until the blood glucose falls to 15 mmol/L. Definite thromboembolic complications require immediate treatment. After treatment, patients should be transferred to subcutaneous insulin injections for a few months; ultimately, most can be controlled with diet or oral antidiabetic agents.

- Transfer to intensive care or high-dependency unit
- Rehydrate with 0.9% isotonic saline with potassium replacement, as for DKA
- Insulin 0.1 units/kg/h or 6 units/h by intravenous infusion.

FIGURE 12.12
Treatment of HONK.

HYPOGLYCAEMIA 13

Hypoglycaemia is a common side-effect of treatment with insulin and some sulphonylurea drugs, and is a major factor preventing type 1 and 2 diabetic patients from achieving near normoglycaemia. The brain is dependent on a continuous supply of glucose, and its interruption for more than a few minutes leads to central nervous system dysfunction, impaired cognition and eventually coma. Hypoglycaemia seems to be associated with sudden death, which usually occurs at night and is apparently caused by cardiac arrhythmias (the 'dead-in-bed syndrome'). Hypoglycaemia is more common in young children and may be responsible for the cognitive impairment and lowered academic achievement in children diagnosed with diabetes under the age of 5 years – the developing brain is especially sensitive to hypoglycaemia. Hypoglycaemia creates as much anxiety among insulin-treated diabetic people as do the long-term complications of blindness and renal failure.

- Obstacle to achieving normoglycaemia
- Disabling symptoms
- Sudden death syndrome
- Cognitive impairment in children
- Major source of anxiety in patients

FIGURE 13.1
Some consequences of hypoglycaemia in diabetes.

During standard insulin therapy in type 1 diabetes, about 10% of patients have at least one severe hypoglycaemic episode in a year. This can increase up to threefold in those treated by intensified insulin injection therapy. In the Diabetes Control and Complications Trial (which compared the effects of intensive and conventional control on diabetic tissue complications in type 1 diabetes), hypoglycaemia increased in proportion to the reduction in glycated haemoglobin. Rates of hypoglycaemia for type 2 diabetes are lower – about 2.5% of insulin-treated and 0.5% per year of sulphonylurea-treated type 2 patients.

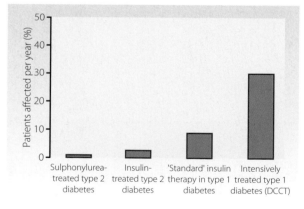

FIGURE 13.2
Risks of severe hypoglycaemia associated with different diabetes treatments.

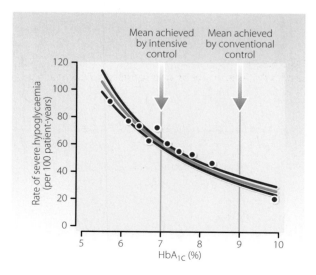

FIGURE 13.3
Relationship between the frequency of severe hypoglycaemia and the quality of glycaemic control, as measured by HbA_{1c}, in the DCCT trial.

Hypoglycaemia in diabetes is caused by inappropriately raised insulin concentrations or enhanced insulin effect, because of excessive insulin dosage (e.g. mismatch of the timing and/or the amount of insulin and food), increased bioavailability (e.g. accelerated absorption in exercise, or reduced clearance in renal failure), increased sensitivity (e.g. counter-regulatory hormone deficiencies, such as in Addison's disease or pituitary failure, or after physical training), and inadequate carbohydrate intake (e.g. missed meals). Other factors include gastroparesis (with its associated vomiting and delayed digestion), alcohol (which inhibits hepatic glucose production) and various drugs (see Chapter 26).

Excessive insulin levels		Enhanced insulin effect		
Excessive dosage	**Increased insulin bioavailability**	**Increased insulin sensitivity**	**Inadequate carbohydrate intake**	**Other factors**
Error by patient, doctor or pharmacist	Accelerated absorption	Counter-regulatory hormone deficiencies	Missed, small or delayed meals	Exercise
Poor matching to patient's needs or lifestyle needs or lifestyle	• Exercise	• Addison's disease	Slimming diets	• Acute: accelerated absorption
	• Injection into abdomen	• Hypopituitarism	Anorexia nervosa	• Late: repletion of muscle glycogen
Deliberate overdose (factitious hypoglycaemia)	• Change to human insulin	Weight loss	Vomiting, including gastroparesis	Alcohol (inhibits hepatic glucose production)
	Insulin antibodies (release of bound insulin)	Physical training	Breast feeding	Drugs
	Renal failure (reduced insulin clearance)	Postpartum	Failure to cover exercise (early or delayed hypoglycaemia)	• Enhance sulphonylurea action (salicylates, sulphonamides)
	'Honeymoon period' (partial β-cell recovery)	Menstrual cycle variation		• Block counter-regulation (non-selective β-blockers)

FIGURE 13.4
Factors that precipitate or predispose to hypoglycaemia.

In the non-diabetic person, hypoglycaemia is limited in part by inhibition of insulin release from the pancreatic β cells and associated stimulation of glucagon secretion from α cells. The major physiological responses to hypoglycaemia follow activation of neurones in the ventromedial region of the hypothalamus and elsewhere in the brain; these sense the lowered glucose levels and activate both the autonomic nervous system and pituitary counter-regulatory hormone release. Glucagon and epinephrine (adrenaline) release are probably the main factors that limit hypoglycaemia and ensure glucose recovery.

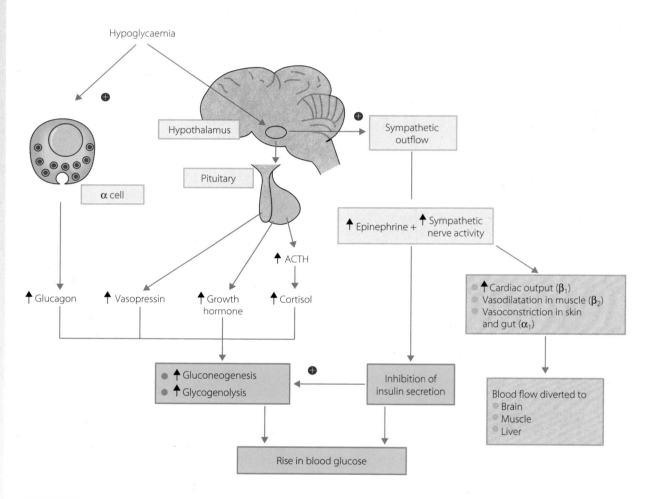

FIGURE 13.5
Major components of the counter-regulatory and sympathetic responses to hypoglycaemia. Vasopressin has weak counter-regulatory effects on its own, but acts synergistically with the other hormones.

The physiological responses to a falling glucose level produce a range of symptoms that help individuals to recognize hypoglycaemia and take corrective action. Hypoglycaemic symptoms can be classified as 'autonomic', caused by the activation of the sympathetic or parasympathetic nervous system (e.g. tremor, palpitations or sweating), or 'neuroglycopenic', caused by the effects of glucose deprivation on the brain (e.g. drowsiness, confusion and loss of consciousness). Headache and nausea are probably non-specific symptoms of malaise. Autonomic symptoms are prominent in subjects with a short duration of diabetes, but diminish with increasing duration.

Autonomic	Neuroglycopenic	Malaise
Sweating	Confusion	Nausea
Pounding heart	Drowsiness	Headache
Shaking (tremor)	Speech difficulty	
Hunger	Incoordination	
	Atypical behaviour	
	Visual disturbance	
	Circumoral paraesthesiae	

FIGURE 13.6
Common symptoms of acute hypoglycaemia in diabetic patients.

The initial response to hypoglycaemia is the acute release of counter-regulatory hormones (most importantly, glucagon and epinephrine) which occurs at a plasma glucose concentration of about 3.6–3.8 mmol/L (65–68 mg/dL). Autonomic symptoms develop at about 3.2 mmol/L (58 mg/dL), before cognitive function starts to deteriorate at around 3 mmol/L (54 mg/dL). Those who retain awareness of hypoglycaemia are thus alerted before significant cerebral dysfunction occurs. However, the inability to recognize impending hypoglycaemia, 'hypoglycaemia unawareness', is a major clinical problem in those with insulin-treated diabetes, and it affects about 25% of those with type 1 diabetes. In these patients, sympathoadrenal activation occurs at a lower glucose level than for cognitive impairment. The risk of a severe episode of hypoglycaemia increases 6–7 fold in those with hypoglycaemia unawareness.

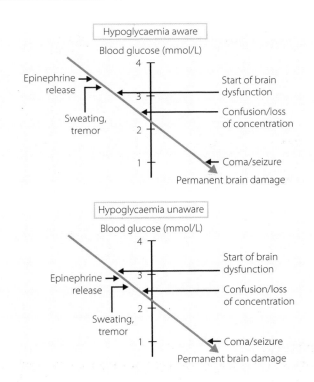

FIGURE 13.7
Glycaemic thresholds for the release of epinephrine and activation of autonomic symptoms and for neuroglycopenic effects in diabetic subjects who are aware or unaware of hypoglycaemia. Note that in those who are unaware of hypoglycaemia, activation of autonomic symptoms occurs at a glycaemic threshold below that for cognitive impairment.

129

Nearly all people with insulin-treated diabetes have some defect in the mechanisms that protect them against hypoglycaemia, although impairment is mild in type 2 diabetes. The glucagon response to hypoglycaemia begins to fail within 1–2 years' duration in those with type 1 diabetes, probably because of disruption of the paracrine insulin cross-talk within the islet, as endogenous insulin production declines. A reduced sympathoadrenal response is common in type 1 diabetes of long duration; those who exhibit both glucagon and epinephrine impairment are particularly susceptible to hypoglycaemia, because of both impaired glucose counter-regulation and impaired hypoglycaemia awareness.

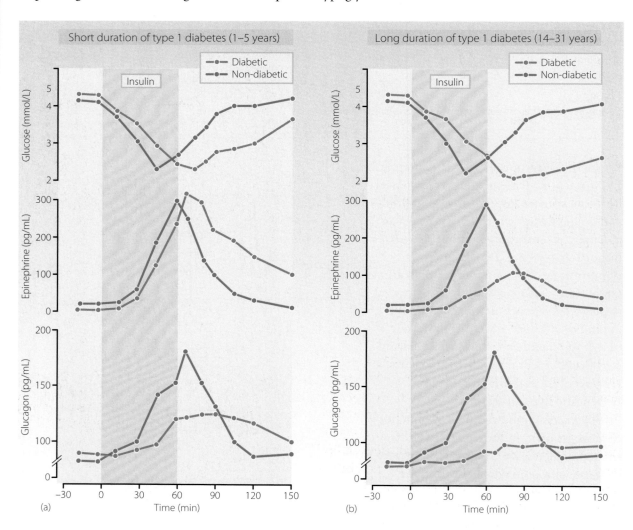

FIGURE 13.8

Impairment of counter-regulatory responses in type 1 diabetes. (a) After 1–5 years of type 1 diabetes, the mean glucagon response (lower panel) is blunted, but the rise in epinephrine secretion is preserved (middle panel) and glycaemic recovery is delayed (upper panel). (b) With long-standing type 1 diabetes, both glucagon and epinephrine responses are impaired severely and glycaemic recovery is markedly delayed and slowed.

HANDBOOK OF DIABETES 3RD EDITION

Severe hypoglycaemia is relatively uncommon in the first few years after diagnosis of diabetes, but increases with diabetes duration in both type 1 and 2 diabetes. Almost 50% of type 1 diabetic subjects with diabetes for more than 20 years have some degree of hypoglycaemia unawareness. The effect of diabetes duration is unexplained, but might involve progressive failure of endogenous insulin production and thus altered glucagon responses, and/or the consequences of repeated hypoglycaemia (see below). Classic autonomic neuropathy (Chapter 17) is thought not to be an important cause of hypoglycaemia unawareness.

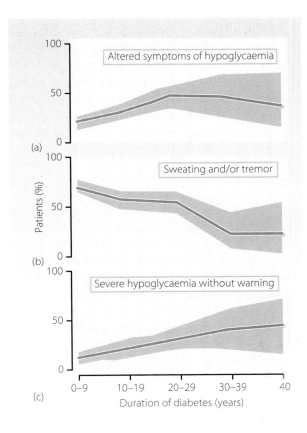

FIGURE 13.9
Relationships between the duration of diabetes and the percentages of 411 diabetic patients who reported changes in symptoms of hypoglycaemia (a); sweating and/or tremor as one of their two cardinal symptoms of hypoglycaemia (b); and severe hypoglycaemia episodes without warning symptoms (c).

A further major factor associated with impaired physiological defences to hypoglycaemia and hypoglycaemia unawareness is strict glycaemic control – which effectively resets thresholds for the counter-regulatory and symptomatic responses to hypoglycaemia at a lower glucose level. Antecedent hypoglycaemia contributes to defective responses to subsequent hypoglycaemia, which leads to a vicious circle of reduced awareness, increased vulnerability and further episodes of hypoglycaemia. It is likely that the neurones that initiate the autonomic response adapt to chronic hypoglycaemia by increasing glucose transporter expression and glucose uptake; subsequent hypoglycaemia fails to produce sufficient intracellular glycopenia and thus no longer elicits a response. There is also evidence that cortisol (released during the counter-regulatory response to hypoglycaemia) dampens the hypothalamic sensing of glucose.

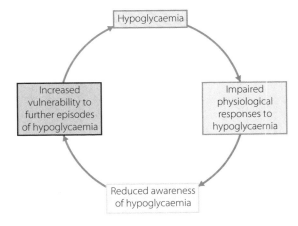

FIGURE 13.10
The vicious circle of repeated hypoglycaemia.

Impaired hormonal responses and hypoglycaemia unawareness can be reversed, at least in part, by strict avoidance of hypoglycaemia. Clinical approaches that may reduce hypoglycaemia include training in insulin-dose adjustment according to frequent blood glucose monitoring, 'blood glucose awareness training' (i.e. teaching patients to recognize all levels of blood glucose using symptoms, performance cues and mood) and the setting of appropriate compromise glycaemic targets (e.g. HbA$_{1c}$ not below 6%). Continuous subcutaneous insulin infusion (CSII, see Chapter 10) is associated with a lower frequency of hypoglycaemia than multiple insulin injection therapy and should be considered as a therapeutic option in those with frequent, unpredictable hypoglycaemia. Modifying intensified insulin regimens – such as using a rapid-acting insulin analogue in a basal-bolus regimen – may also decrease the risk of hypoglycaemia.

- Frequent contact between patient and health-care professional
- Regular blood glucose monitoring
- Nocturnal blood glucose measurement
- Avoidance of all hypoglycaemic episodes
- Glucose targets that prevent biochemical hypoglycaemia
- Consider CSII

FIGURE 13.11
Important features of a hypoglycaemia-avoidance programme

Suspected severe hypoglycaemia (e.g. in a diabetic patient with impaired consciousness or coma) should be confirmed if possible by blood glucose testing (reagent strips). It should be treated immediately with oral glucose or, if the patient is unconscious or unable to swallow safely, with intravenous glucose or intramuscular or subcutaneous glucagon injection. Patients usually recover within minutes.

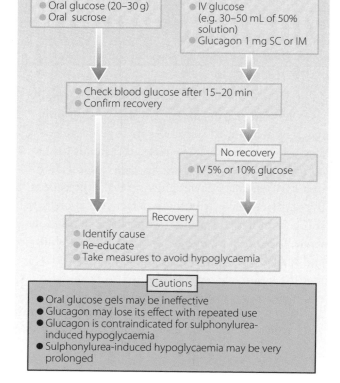

FIGURE 13.12
Algorithm for treating acute hypoglycaemia in diabetic patients. Some important cautions are also indicated.

Much of the impact of chronic diabetes results from the development of tissue complications, mainly microvascular disease (microangiopathy, retinopathy, nephropathy and neuropathy) and macrovascular disease (atherosclerosis). Microangiopathy is characterized by progressive occlusion of the vascular lumen with impaired perfusion, increased vascular permeability and increased elaboration of extracellular material by perivascular cells, which results in basement membrane thickening. There is strong evidence that microvascular disease is related to the duration and severity of hyperglycaemia in both type 1 and type 2 diabetes. A classic observational study by Pirart demonstrated this link in 4400 type 1 and 2 patients followed up for up to 25 years. As diabetes duration increased, the prevalence of retinopathy, nephropathy and neuropathy was highest in those with poor glycaemic control and lowest in those with good control.

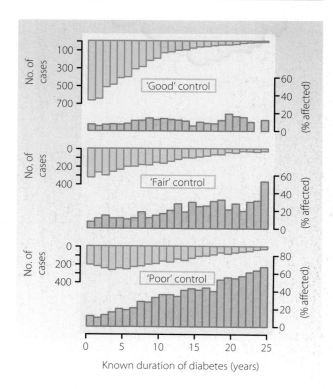

FIGURE 14.1
Prevalence of diabetic neuropathy as a function of duration of diabetes in patients with 'good', 'fair' and 'poor' control.

Many other epidemiological studies support this relationship. In the Wisconsin Epidemiologic Study of Diabetic Retinopathy (WESDR), a population study of diabetic people living in and receiving their primary medical care in the state of Wisconsin (USA), the incidence and progression of retinopathy in type 1 ('younger onset') and type 2 ('older onset') diabetic subjects was clearly related to glycaemic status.

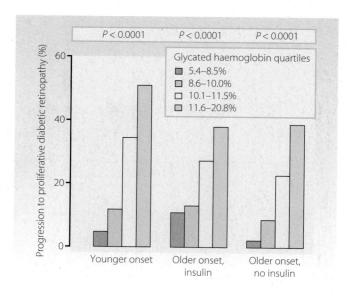

FIGURE 14.2
Progression of proliferative retinopathy is related to glycated haemoglobin percentage in the Wisconsin Eye Study.

Convincing proof of the 'glucose hypothesis' for complications in type 1 diabetes came with the Diabetes Control and Complications Trial (DCCT, reported in 1993). This trial is often regarded as a landmark in diabetes research; 1440 patients at 29 centres in North America were allocated randomly to either 'conventional' therapy (one or two daily insulin injections, 3-monthly clinic visits, no insulin dosage adjustments according to self-monitored glucose data), or to 'intensive' therapy [three or more daily insulin injections or insulin pump therapy (CSII), monthly clinic visits and weekly telephone calls, frequent blood glucose self monitoring with insulin dosage adjustment, and a diet and exercise programme]. Throughout the 9-year study, there was markedly better glycaemic control in the intensively treated group.

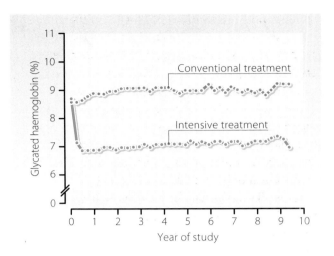

FIGURE 14.3
Glycaemic control achieved in the DCCT.

Clinically important retinopathy, nephropathy (urinary albumin excretion) and neuropathy were substantially reduced in the strict control group. For example, the cumulative frequency of retinopathy in those without this complication at the start of the study ('primary prevention' cohort) was reduced by about 75% in the intensively treated patients. In those with early retinopathy at baseline ('secondary prevention' cohort), the average risk of progression was reduced by about 50%.

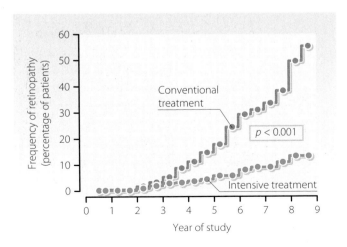

FIGURE 14.4
Beneficial effect of intensive treatment on the onset of retinopathy. Cumulative incidence of background retinopathy in type 1 diabetic patients who entered the DCCT without retinopathy.

HANDBOOK OF DIABETES 3RD EDITION

Analogous randomized controlled trial evidence for the role of glycaemic control in microvascular disease in type 2 diabetes comes from the United Kingdom Prospective Diabetes Study (UKPDS, reported in 1998). This 20-year study recruited over 5000 type 2 diabetic patients in 23 centres throughout the UK. In the main study, 3867 newly diagnosed type 2 patients were allocated randomly to either so-called 'intensive' therapy (the sulphonylureas, chlorpropamide, glibenclamide or glipizide, or to insulin) or to 'conventional' therapy, which was diet initially, though tablets or insulin could be added later if symptoms or marked hyperglycaemia developed. Over 10 years, there was a reduction in HbA_{1c} from 7.9 to 7.0% with intensive treatment, though in both groups glycaemic control deteriorated throughout the study. Intensive therapy in these type 2 diabetic subjects was associated with a significant 25% reduction in microvascular disease endpoints.

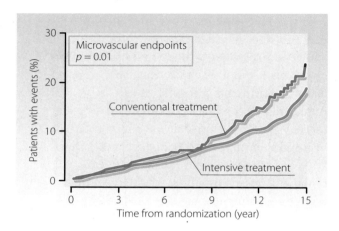

FIGURE 14.5
Effect of intensive blood glucose control on microvascular complications in type 2 diabetes (UKPDS).

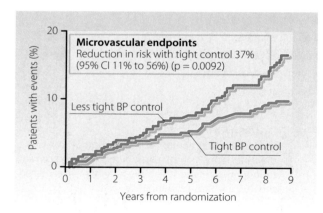

`FIGURE 14.6
Kaplan–Meier plots of proportions of patients who developed microvascular endpoints (mostly retinal photocoagulation) during tight or less tight BP control (UKPDS).

There are exceptions to the rule that the quality of diabetic control determines microvascular complications (e.g. a few patients with relatively mild hyperglycaemia can develop severe microangiopathy). It seems that individual susceptibility to glucose-induced tissue damage is influenced by other factors. One of the most important of these is blood pressure. This was clearly demonstrated in the UKPDS trial, in which 1148 hypertensive patients with type 2 diabetes were allocated to either tight or less tight control of blood pressure (mean BP over 9 years 144/82 vs 154/87 mmHg). Microvascular endpoints were reduced by 37% in the group with the lower blood pressure.

HANDBOOK OF DIABETES 3RD EDITION

An intriguing feature of diabetic microangiopathy is 'hyperglycaemic memory' (i.e. progression of microvascular disease even though diabetic control has been improved significantly). In the DCCT, there was a latent period of about 4 years before tightly controlled patients began to show improvement. Conversely, when the DCCT ended, diabetic control relaxed in previously strictly controlled patients; in these cases, the slowed evolution of microangiopathy persisted for some 4 years – even though post-trial glycaemic control was nearly identical to that in the patients who had been treated conventionally during the trial.

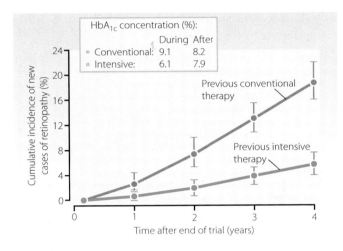

FIGURE 14.7
'Hyperglycaemic memory'. After the end of the DCCT study, the group that had been poorly controlled on conventional insulin therapy continued to suffer a higher incidence of diabetic retinopathy than did the tightly controlled group given intensive therapy, even though post-trial glycaemic control was comparable in the two groups.

Epidemiological studies also show a clear positive relationship between glycaemia and macrovascular disease in the *general* population. For example, in the European Prospective Investigation of Cancer and Nutrition (EPIC) study of 4600 men in East Anglia, UK, HbA_{1c} was continuously related to cardiovascular mortality from the lowest level below 5% to values >7% and in self-reported diabetes. However, it is generally believed that the duration and degree of hyperglycaemia have a much less important role in the causation of diabetic macroangiopathy than they do in microangiopathy (see Chapter 20). Both the DCCT and UKPDS provide only borderline support for any significant reduction in macrovascular disease in diabetes by the improving glycaemic control. Other factors, such as hypertension, hyperlipidaemia and smoking (the 'bad companions'), conspire with hyperglycaemia to promote diabetic macrovascular disease.

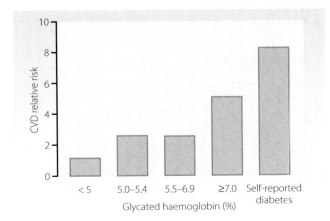

FIGURE 14.8
The relationship between glycated haemoglobin percentage and cardiovascular disease (CVD) in the EPIC Norfolk Study of 4662 men.

HANDBOOK OF DIABETES 3RD EDITION

Diabetes particularly affects tissues that cannot downregulate glucose uptake when extracellular glucose increases, leading to raised intracellular glucose concentrations. One mechanism by which hyperglycaemia may cause complications is by an increased flux of glucose through the polyol pathway. In this pathway, the rate-limiting enzyme, aldose reductase, reduces glucose to its sugar alcohol, sorbitol. Sorbitol is then oxidized by sorbitol dehydrogenase into fructose. Aldose reductase is found in tissues such as nerve, the retina, the glomerulus and the blood vessel wall, where glucose uptake is independent of GLUT-4 and insulin. The pathway is normally inactive because of the high K_m of aldose reductase, but hyperglycaemia increases flux through the pathway and leads to accumulation of intracellular glucose and glucose-derived substances, such as methylglyoxal and acetol (which rapidly glycate proteins). Sorbitol does not diffuse easily across cell membranes and damage may occur because of sorbitol-induced osmotic stress (currently thought to be less likely). Alternative mechanisms may involve decreased NADPH, thereby decreasing reduced glutathione, an important scavenger of reactive oxygen species; or an increased NADH/NAD$^+$ ratio, which inhibits glyceraldehyde 3-phosphate dehydrogenase, increasing intracellular triose phosphate and the formation of methylglyoxal and activation of protein kinase C (see below).

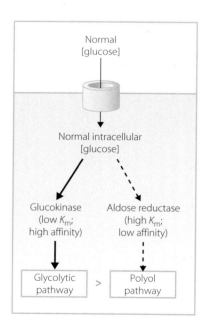
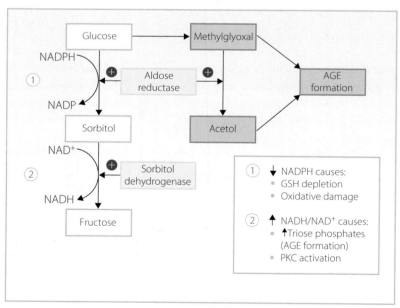

FIGURE 14.9

The polyol pathway. *Left*: The pathway is normally inactive, but becomes active when intracellular glucose levels rise. *Right*: Consequences of increased glucose flux through the polyol pathway include the generation of powerful glycating sugars (methylglyoxal, acetol and triose phosphates), enhanced oxidative damage and protein kinase C (PKC) activation. AGE, advanced glycation end-products; GSH, reduced glutathione; NAD, nicotinamide adenine dinucleotide.

Another mechanism for glucose damage is thought to be increased intracellular formation of advanced glycation end-products (AGEs). AGEs are formed by the reaction of glucose and other glycating compounds, such as methylglyoxal with proteins (compare the formation of glycated haemoglobin, Chapter 9), and other long-lived molecules, such nucleic acids. Early glycation products are reversible, but eventually they undergo irreversible changes through cross-linking, which impairs protein structure and function.

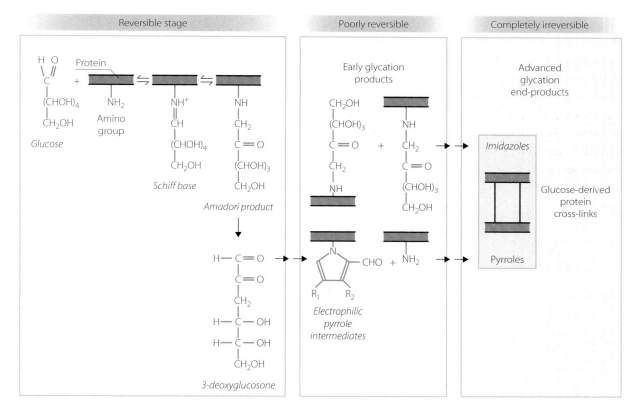

FIGURE 14.10
Formation of reversible, early, non-enzymatic glycation products, and of irreversible advanced glycation end-products (AGEs). Through a complex series of chemical reactions, Amadori products can form families of imidazole-based and pyrrole-based glucose-derived cross-links.

GE can damage cells by altering cellular protein function and by cross-linking extracellular matrix molecules, such as collagen and laminin, which in the blood vessels increases wall thickness and permeability, and decreases elasticity. AGE-modified circulating proteins bind to specific receptors (RAGEs) on several types of cell, including monocyte/macrophages, glomerular mesangial cells and endothelial cells. This binding leads to the generation of reactive oxygen species, activation of the transcription factor NFκB and stimulation of cytokine and growth factor production, inflammatory cell adhesion (via increased VCAM-1), procoagulant protein expression and increased vascular permeability (e.g. via vascular endothelial growth factor, VEGF).

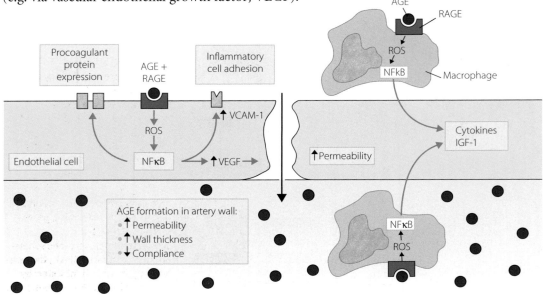

FIGURE 14.11

Possible mechanisms of cell damage by interactions of advanced glycation end-products (AGEs) with their receptor (RAGE) in endothelial cells and macrophages. IGF, insulin-like growth factor; NFκB, nuclear factor kappa B; ROS, reactive oxygen species; VCAM-1, vascular cell adhesion molecule-1; VEGF, vascular endothelium-derived growth factor.

rotein kinase C (PKC) is an enzyme that phosphorylates several target proteins. It exists in several isoforms and is activated by diacylglycerol. Excessive activation of PKC is a further mechanism by which glucose might induce tissue damage, since diacylglycerol is formed *de novo* from glucose *via* triose phosphates in the glycolytic pathway. Overactivity of PKC has been implicated in increased vascular permeability, blood flow changes and increased basement membrane synthesis. Some of the effects may be mediated by PKC's inhibition of nitric oxide (NO) production.

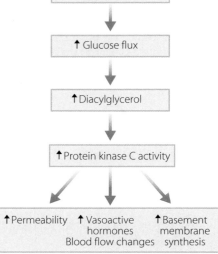

FIGURE 14.12

Activation of protein kinase C by *de-novo* synthesis of diacylglycerol, following increased glucose utilization.

Hyperglycaemia might also cause diabetic complications by shunting glucose into the hexosamine pathway. Here, fructose-6-phosphate is diverted from glycolysis to form UDP-*N*-acetylglucosamine, used in the synthesis of glycoproteins. The rate-limiting step in the conversion of glucose to glucosamine is regulated by glutamine:fructose-6-phosphate amidotransferase (GFAT). Possibly, glycation of transcription factors by *N*-acetylglucosamine increases the transcription of key genes such as TGF-β, acetyl CoA carboxylase (the rate-limiting enzyme for fatty acid synthesis), plasminogen activator inhibitor-1 (PAI-1) and probably many other genes.

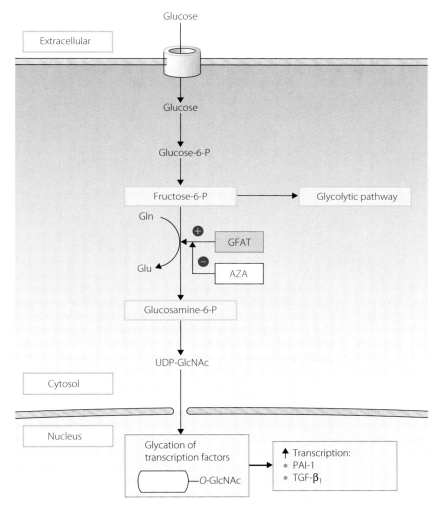

FIGURE 14.13
The glucosamine pathway. Glucosamine-6-phosphate, generated from fructose-6-phosphate and glutamine (Gln), is converted into UDP-*N*-acetylglucosamine (UDP-GlcNAc), which can glycate transcription factors and thus enhance transcription of genes including plasminogen activator inhibitor (PAI)-1 and transforming growth factor-β_1 (TGF-β_1). Glutamine:fructose-6-phosphate amidotransferase (GFAT), the rate-limiting enzyme, is inhibited by azaserine (AZA). Glu, glutamic acid.

All four of the above mechanisms might result from glucose-induced mitochondrial overproduction of superoxide. This stimulates aldose reductase activity, enhances methylglyoxal synthesis and thus AGE, increases diacylglycerol and PKC activation, and activates the hexosamine pathway.

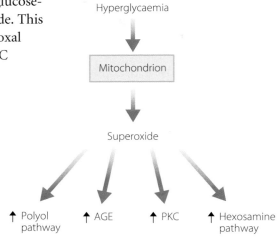

FIGURE 14.14
Superoxide links glucose excess and diabetic complications.

Diabetic eye disease primarily affects the retinal blood vessels, but diabetes also accelerates cataract formation (lens opacities). The clinically observable lesions of diabetic retinopathy can be grouped into categories, according to the features seen on ophthalmoscopy – background, preproliferative and proliferative retinopathy, and maculopathy. There are several similar schemes for grading the severity of retinopathy, including the Early Treatment of Diabetic Retinopathy (ETDRS) grading, which is widely used in North America, and the UK National Guidelines on Screening for Diabetic Retinopathy system.

Background (Level 1)
- Microaneurysm(s)
- Retinal haemorrhage(s) ± any exudates

Preproliferative (Level 2)
- Venous beading
- Venous loop or reduplication
- IRMA
- Multiple deep, round haemorrhages
- Cotton-wool spots

Proliferative (Level 3)
- New vessels on disc (NVD)
- New vessels elsewhere (NVE)
- Preretinal or vitreous haemorrhage
- Preretinal fibrosis ± tractional retinal detatchment

Maculopathy
- Exudate within a disc area (DA) of fovea
- Retinal thickening within DA of fovea
- Microaneurysm or haemorrhage within DA of fovea

FIGURE 15.1
The lesions of diabetic retinopathy and a simplified grading (UK National Guidelines on Screening for Diabetic Retinopathy).

Early subclinical abnormalities of the retinal vessels are thickening of the basement membrane, loss of pericytes (the contractile cells that control vessel calibre and flow), increased blood flow and increased capillary permeability.

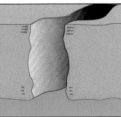

Pericyte

Endothelium

Basement membrane

FIGURE 15.2
Structure of the retinal microvasculature. The endothelial cells are normally joined by tight junctions, which constitute much of the blood–retinal barrier; these separate in diabetes, causing increased vascular permeability. Other abnormalities in diabetes include thickening of the basement membrane and fallout of both the endothelial cells and the contractile pericytes.

Tight junction

Adherens junction

Basement membrane

Normal

Diabetic

Background retinopathy is the first stage of retinopathy and is not associated with visual loss unless the macula becomes involved (maculopathy). Microaneurysms are the earliest clinical sign of retinopathy and appear as small red dots, which vary in size from about 20 to 200 µm. They are blind outgrowths of the retinal capillaries and develop where the wall is weakened (perhaps because of pericyte loss) or adjacent to areas of capillary non-perfusion. They are more obvious as white dots on fluorescein angiography (fluorescein injected intravenously binds to albumin; when photographed under ultraviolet light, the technique reveals retinal anatomy, together with areas of vascular leakage, microaneurysms and new vessels). Individual microaneurysms come and go.

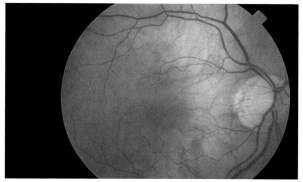

FIGURE 15.3
Microaneurysms: the earliest sign of diabetic retinopathy. This is a myopic eye with a pale fundus.

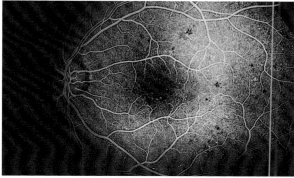

FIGURE 15.4
Fluorescein angiogram, showing microaneurysms as small white dots and haemorrhages as larger black spots.

Haemorrhages are another feature of background retinopathy; they tend to be flame shaped when they occur superficially or round (blot shaped) when they lie deeper in the retina. Larger 'blot' haemorrhages are associated with retinal ischaemia. Hard exudates result from the deposition of lipid-rich proteins within the retina as a result of capillary leakage. They appear as yellowish white opacities, which are often ring shaped (circinate) when there is a focus of leakage (as in focal diabetic maculopathy).

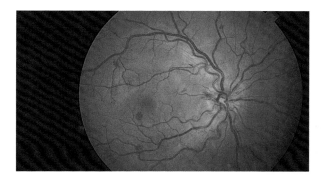

FIGURE 15.5
Retinal haemorrhages: red 'blots'.

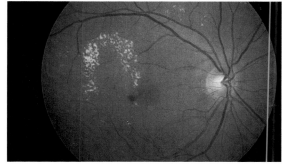

FIGURE 15.6
Focal diabetic maculopathy with circinate (ring-shaped) exudate. Laser treatment is applied to the leaking microaneurysms at the centre of the circinate exudates.

Preproliferative retinopathy is caused by worsening retinal ischaemia and carries a high risk of developing into sight-threatening proliferative retinopathy. Preproliferative changes include multiple (>5 per eye) cotton-wool spots (i.e. fluffy white spots caused by the accumulation of intracellular axoplasmic material that results from infarcts in the nerve fibre layer).

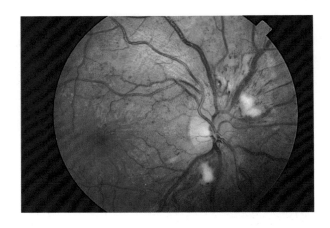

FIGURE 15.7
Cotton-wool spots around the optic disc.

Intraretinal microvascular abnormalities (IRMAs) are clusters of irregular, branched vessels in the retina, which may represent attempts at neovascularization. Like cotton-wool spots and large blot haemorrhages, they are associated with extensive retinal ischaemia. Venous changes in preproliferative retinopathy may include beading (segmental dilatations, like a string of sausages), loops and reduplication.

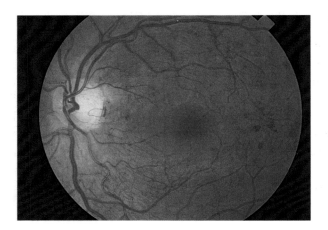

FIGURE 15.8
IRMAs.

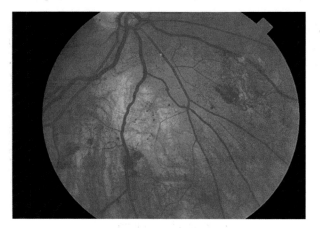

FIGURE 15.9
Venous irregularity or 'beading' (centre of field) and new vessels elsewhere (NVE, top right of field).

Proliferative retinopathy is marked by abnormal new vessels (neovascularization), stimulated by growth factors (e.g. vascular endothelium-derived growth factor, VEGF) released from the ischaemic retina. New vessels are very fine, branching vessels that arise from retinal veins and grow forward towards the vitreous and overlie the other retinal vessels. New vessels on the disc (NVD) carry the highest risk of progression to severe sight loss.

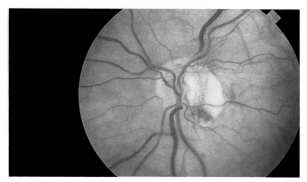

FIGURE 15.10
More extensive new vessels on the disc (NVD), occupying more than half the disc diameter.

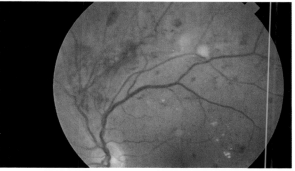

FIGURE 15.11
Extensive new vessels elsewhere (NVE) above the disc, with widespread signs of retinal ischaemia.

New vessels are always associated with the development of fibrous tissue, appearing as a grey–white membrane, which persists even after treatment. Sometimes this may contract, leading to retinal detachment or avulsion of vessels where they enter the vitreous gel, causing a vitreous haemorrhage. Vitreous haemorrhage causes sudden loss of vision and, on ophthalmoscopy, obscures retinal detail.

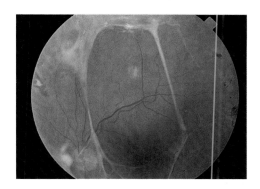

FIGURE 15.12
Fibrous bands that are exerting traction on the retina. The retinal scars are from previous xenon laser treatment.

Haemorrhage into the space between the gel and the retina (preretinal) may remain encapsulated, when sedimentation of uncoagulated blood results in a flat-topped ('boat-shaped') appearance.

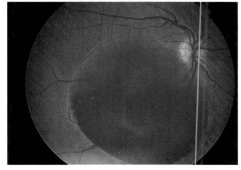

FIGURE 15.13
Preretinal haemorrhage. Note the settling of the uncoagulated blood.

In tractional retinal detachment, the retina appears distorted and lifted into greyish white folds with associated tears. Ultrasonography can be used to diagnose retinal detachment when the view of the fundus is obscured by a vitreous haemorrhage.

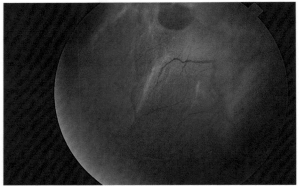

FIGURE 15.14
Rhegmatogenous retinal detachment: a large retinal tear (red lesion) is present at 12 o'clock, and the detached retina appears grey and folded.

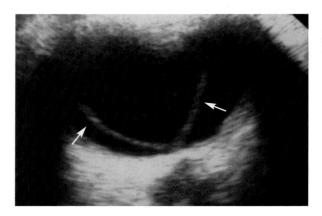

FIGURE 15.15
B-scan ultrasound image of the eye, showing a retinal detachment that was invisible behind a dense vitreous haemorrhage.

Sight can also be threatened by glaucoma caused by neovascular tissue on the iris and at the drainage angle (rubeosis iridis). Glaucoma is more likely in eyes that have had cataract surgery or vitrectomy, especially when retinal laser photocoagulation has not been performed or is incomplete. Neovascular glaucoma is extremely unpleasant and can lead to a painful blind eye.

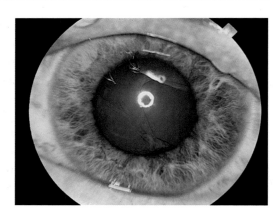

FIGURE 15.16
New vessels on the iris (rubeosis iridis). There is also a vitreous haemorrhage.

Maculopathy results from retinal oedema and thickening close to the macula, and can threaten or cause loss of central vision. Focal maculopathy consists of retinal oedema within one disc diameter of the macula centre, and is often associated with hard exudates around the area of leakage, typically circinate (in a ring) or radiating outwards (macular 'star'). More diffuse maculopathy may be difficult to recognize without stereoscopic examination (which reveals retinal thickening). Maculopathy is most common in type 2 diabetes and can cause severe visual loss.

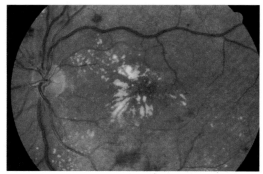

FIGURE 15.17
Diffuse macular oedema, with a macular 'star'. This requires grid laser photocoagulation.

Cataract is a common cause of blindness in diabetic patients. It is recognized as an opacity against the red fundal reflex when the eye is examined with an ophthalmoscope at a distance of 30 cm. The mechanisms of normal age-related and irreversible diabetic cataract are probably similar. Non-enzymatic glycation and subsequent cross-linking of the lens protein (α-crystallin) probably contribute. Also, sorbitol accumulation in the diabetic lens could lead to osmotic swelling, although evidence for this mechanism in humans is less strong than in experimental diabetic cataracts in other species.

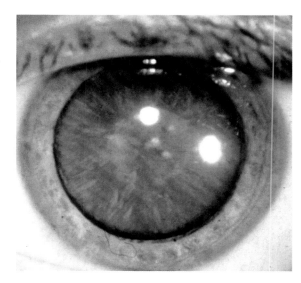

FIGURE 15.18
Diabetic cataract.

Regular examination of the eyes in the diabetic patient is essential and should include visual acuity measurement with a Snellen chart (uncorrected and corrected with spectacles or pinhole) and examination of the fundus through dilated pupils. In recent years, digital fundus photography has been introduced as a regular screening tool in many diabetic clinics. It provides permanent records that can be examined later by the ophthalmologist or trained non-clinical assessor. Yearly examinations are recommended for those with no retinopathy, 6-monthly for those with background retinopathy and referral to an ophthalmologist when the retina is obscured by cataract or haemorrhage, and for specific clinical problems, such as sudden loss of vision or unexplained drop in visual acuity, retinal detachment, new vessel formation, vitreous or preretinal haemorrhage, maculopathy and pre- or severe non-proliferative retinopathy.

Clinical problem	Urgency of referral
Sudden loss of vision	Within 1 day
Evidence of retinal detachment	Within 1 day
New vessel formation (on the disc or elsewhere)	Within 1 week
Vitreous or preretinal haemorrhage	Within 1 week
Rubeosis iridis	Within 1 week
Hard exudates within 1 DD of the fovea	Within 4 weeks
Clinically significant macular oedema	Within 4 weeks
Unexplained drop in visual acuity	Within 4 weeks
Unexplained retinal findings	Within 4 weeks
Severe or very severe non-proliferative retinopathy	Within 4 weeks

FIGURE 15.19
Diabetic retinopathy referral guidelines for specialist assessment.

HANDBOOK OF DIABETES 3RD EDITION

Panretinal photocoagulation is used to treat new vessels and preproliferative retinopathy. Large areas of the peripheral retina are ablated by the patterned application of 500 µm laser burns. This concentrates the blood supply on the remaining retina and diminishes the ischaemic stimulus to new vessel formation. Regression of neovascularization is often achieved with a total of 1200–1500 burns in two or three treatment sessions, and may hold further neovascularization at bay thereafter.

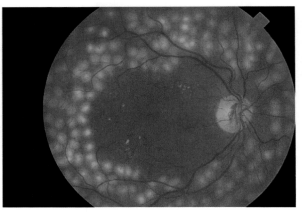

FIGURE 15.20
Fresh panretinal (scatter) laser photocoagulation burns for treating new vessels on the disc.

Laser photocoagulation is also used to treat maculopathy: the laser burns seal leaking vessels, which reduces oedema and the deposition of hard exudates. The 3-year risk of severe visual loss in maculopathy is reduced by over 50% with photocoagulation. The potential side-effects of laser treatment are pain (especially with retreatment – regional anaesthesia is helpful), transient visual loss (associated with retinal bleaching and causing darkening of vision for a few hours), visual field loss, reduced visual acuity (especially with extensive treatment) and choroidal damage leading to haemorrhage and effusion.

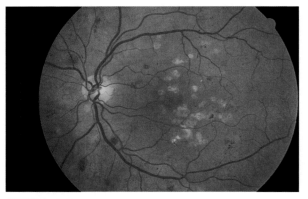

FIGURE 15.21
Focal laser photocoagulation scars around the macula following successful focal treatment.

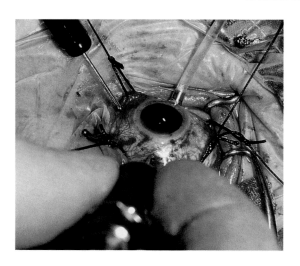

Closed vitreoretinal surgery *via* the pars plana (an avascular area between the anterior edge of the retina and the ciliary body) is used to remove vitreous haemorrhage and fibroproliferative tissue, replace detached retina and repair retinal tears. This surgery can restore and maintain useful vision in up to 70% of eyes with advanced diabetic eye disease.

FIGURE 15.22
Vitrectomy, using common-gauge instruments inserted through the pars plana. Saline is infused through a cannula (top right) to maintain intraocular pressure; vitreous and contained haemorrhage is being disrupted with a cutter (bottom), illuminated by a fibre-optic light source (top left).

- Strict glycaemic control
- Strict blood pressure control
- ACE inhibitors
- Early detection
- Prompt treatment
- Education

FIGURE 15.23
Reducing the risk of diabetic retinopathy.

The results of the DCCT and UKPDS trials show the importance of both strict glycaemic and blood pressure control in reducing the risk of developing retinopathy (see Chapter 14). The anti-hypertensive angiotensin converting enzyme (ACE) inhibitors also reduce the progression of retinopathy (and proteinuria, see Chapter 16) even in normotensive diabetic patients, and are increasingly used, particularly in those with microvascular disease.

Diabetic retinopathy remains one of the most common causes of visual loss in people of working age in the developed world.

DIABETIC NEPHROPATHY   16

The diabetic kidney shows pathological changes in both the glomerulus and the tubular interstitium. At diagnosis of diabetes, the glomerulus is enlarged because of the increased capillary surface area; subsequently, glomerular enlargement is caused by basement membrane thickening and (usually) expansion of the mesangium (the cells and matrix material that support the capillary tufts). Total kidney volume is also increased, mainly through expansion of tubular tissue. Pathological tubular changes include basement membrane thickening, atrophy, interstitial fibrosis and arteriosclerosis. Early in diabetes, the glomerular filtration rate (GFR) is increased because of the increased filtration area, but later the GFR declines in parallel with mesangial expansion and the resultant glomerular occlusion.

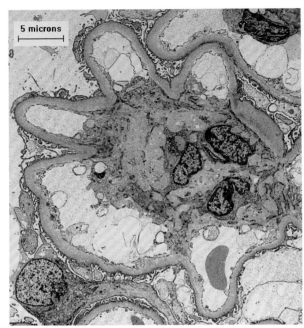

FIGURE 16.1
Electron micrograph of the glomerulus from a diabetic patient, showing basement membrane thickening and mesangial expansion with extracellular matrix accumulation.

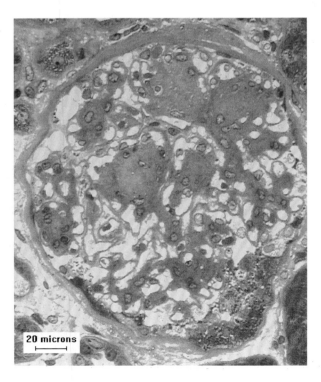

With progression of the disease, mesangial expansion occasionally presents with a structured nodular appearance. These Kimmelstiel–Wilson nodules stain with periodic acid–Schiff reagent and are pathognomonic of diabetic nephropathy.

FIGURE 16.2
Nodular glomerulosclerosis (Kimmelstiel–Wilson kidney) in a patient with diabetic nephropathy.

The natural history of diabetic nephropathy is marked by increasing loss of protein (mostly albumin) in the urine (proteinuria). The initial stage of 'normoalbuminuria' progresses to a phase of incipient nephropathy marked by 'microalbuminuria', in which the increased urinary albumin excretion can be measured only by sensitive immunoassay, and ultimately to dip-stick-positive proteinuria ('clinical' or 'overt' proteinuria). Proteinuria only rarely reaches levels (>3.5 g/day) that cause the nephrotic syndrome. Progression may stop at any stage and can occasionally regress.

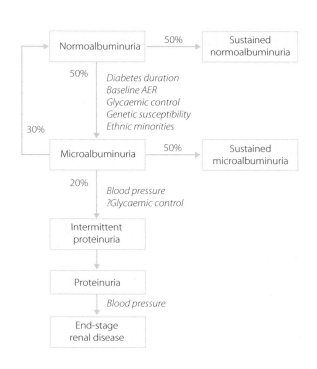

FIGURE 16.3
The stages and determinants of diabetic nephropathy. AER, albumin excretion rate.

Proteinuria is associated with a high mortality. About two-thirds of proteinuric diabetic patients develop terminal renal failure. The rest die from cardiovascular disease. All stages of nephropathy are associated with a greatly increased risk of cardiovascular disease: about 2–3 fold for microalbuminuria and 10 fold for overt proteinuria.

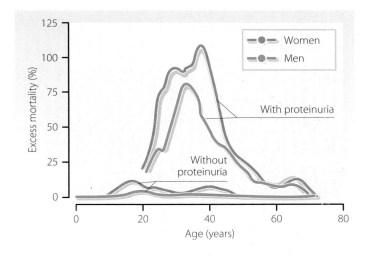

FIGURE 16.4
Relative mortality of diabetic patients with and without persistent proteinuria in men and women as a function of age. Mortality is greatly increased at all ages in proteinuric patients.

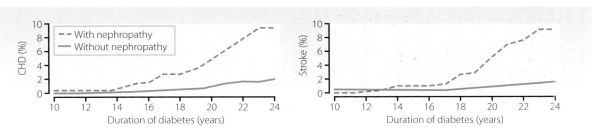

FIGURE 16.5
Cumulative incidence of stroke and coronary heart disease (CHD) in 4702 type 1 diabetic subjects with and without diabetic nephropathy.

Hypertension also affects virtually all patients with persistent proteinuria (>140/90 mmHg in >80%). There are also subtle elevations of blood pressure, even in those patients with microalbuminuria. Diabetic nephropathy is usually accompanied by other clinical problems, in addition to cardiovascular disease and hypertension, principally severe retinopathy, neuropathy and hyperlipidaemia.

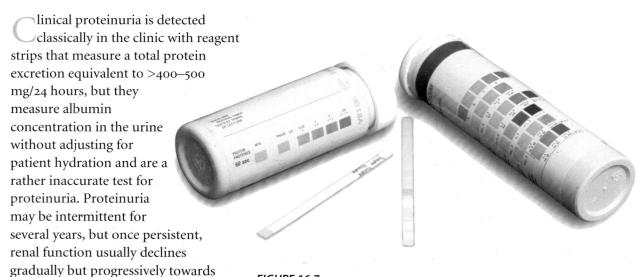

FIGURE 16.6
Prevalence of hypertension in all type 1 diabetic patients (red), in the Danish general population (yellow) and in normoalbuminuric patients (green). DM, diabetes mellitus.

Clinical proteinuria is detected classically in the clinic with reagent strips that measure a total protein excretion equivalent to >400–500 mg/24 hours, but they measure albumin concentration in the urine without adjusting for patient hydration and are a rather inaccurate test for proteinuria. Proteinuria may be intermittent for several years, but once persistent, renal function usually declines gradually but progressively towards end-stage renal failure.

FIGURE 16.7
Dip-stick proteinuria detectable with reagent strips.

Proteinuria is best quantitated by measuring albumin excretion rate in timed urine collections, but for clinical purposes calculation of the albumin:creatinine ratio (ACR) in an early morning urine sample is sufficient, simpler and widely used in diabetic clinics. The categories of proteinuria are at least partly based on renal risk. The actual cut-off values differ somewhat between centres and investigators; a consensus definition of microalbuminuria is 20–200 μg/min in a timed overnight urine sample, 30–300 mg/24 h in a 24-hour collection and 3.5–30 mg/mmol (2.5–30 mg/mmol for females) for ACR.

	Albumin: creatinine ratio (mg/mmol)	Overnight urine collection (μg/min)	24-h urine collection (mg/24 h)
Normoalbuminuria			
Female	< 2.5	< 20	< 30
Male	< 3.5		
Microalbuminuria			
Female	2.5–30	20–200	30–300
Male	3.5–30		
Proteinuria			
Female	> 30	> 200	> 300
Male	> 30		

FIGURE 16.8
Definitions of abnormal urinary albumin excretion.

Early microalbuminuria is probably caused by an increase in transglomerular pressure. As albuminuria worsens, progressive alterations of the glomerular filtration barrier occur, initially with loss of negative charge on the basement membrane and epithelial (podocyte) foot processes, which thus reduces the charge repulsion between the membrane and the polyanionic albumin molecule. Later, macroalbuminuria supervenes when the pore size enlarges, possible secondary to podocyte loss. With advancing renal failure, tubular damage develops and the proteinuria is of mixed glomerular and tubular type.

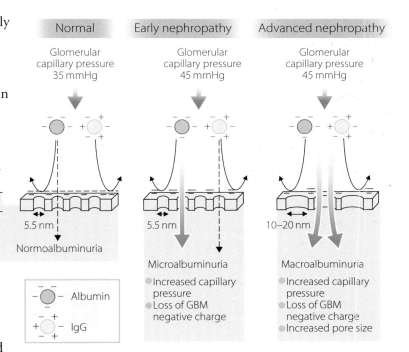

FIGURE 16.9
The evolution of proteinuria in diabetes. GBM, glomerular basement membrane.

The factors most closely associated with progression of diabetic renal disease are diabetes duration, poor glycaemic control, hypertension and baseline albumin excretion rate. Both the Diabetes Control and Complications Trial (DCCT) in type 1 diabetes and the UK Prospective Diabetes Study (UKPDS) in type 2 diabetes demonstrated that improved glycaemic control reduces the risk of microalbuminuria developing. Both studies showed a continuous reduction in microalbuminuria with decreasing HbA_{1c}, without any threshold effect.

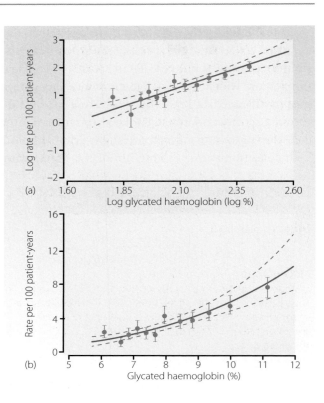

FIGURE 16.10
The absolute risk of microalbuminuria (hazard rate per 100 patient-years) in the combined (intensive and conventional) treatment groups as a function of the updated mean HbA_{1c} during follow-up in the DCCT. (a) Log(rate) vs log(HbA_{1c}). (b) Rate vs HbA_{1c} over the range observed in the trial.

In the UKPDS, tight blood pressure control (mean 144/82 mmHg) resulted in a 29% reduction in the risk of microalbuminuria developing, compared with less stringent blood pressure control (mean 154/87 mmHg). There is particularly good evidence of hypertension in the progression of microalbuminuria and overt proteinuria (see also below). Albumin excretion rate can be reduced by an average of about 50% by 2 years treatment with ACE inhibitors, the usual first-line choice of anti-hypertensive. The effect is greatest in those patients with the highest initial albumin excretion.

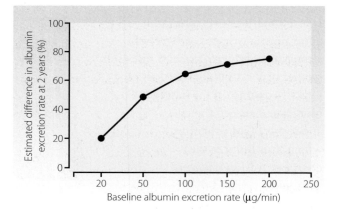

FIGURE 16.11
Meta-analysis of the effects of angiotensin-converting enzyme (ACE) inhibition on microalbuminuria. Estimated difference in albumin excretion rate between placebo and ACE inhibitor treatment groups at 2 years, according to albuminuric status at baseline.

HANDBOOK OF DIABETES 3RD EDITION

About 30% of patients with microalbuminuria revert to normal albumin excretion, while 20% progress to clinical proteinuria, but the risk of developing proteinuria and death remains much greater in those with microalbuminuria at the outset. About 25% of Caucasian type 1 and 2 diabetic patients will develop proteinuria after 25 years of diabetes, but the frequency may be decreasing as the management of diabetes improves. The rates are higher, and may not be improving, in some ethnic groups with high prevalences of diabetes (e.g. UK Asians and Pima Indians in the USA).

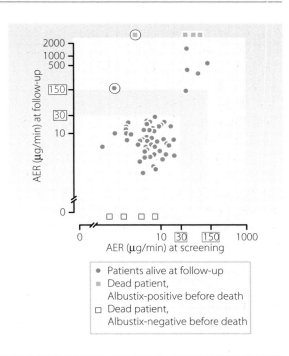

FIGURE 16.12
Outcome after 14 years' follow-up in type 1 diabetic patients with different levels of microalbuminuria at presentation. Most of those with overt proteinuria at follow-up had an albumin excretion rate >30·mg/min at presentation. AER, albumin excretion rate.

Hyperglycaemia may cause renal damage through several mechanisms, including non-enzymatic glycation of proteins, activation of the polyol pathway, activation of the hexosamine pathway and increased intracellular reactive oxygen species (see Chapter 14). Although hyperglycaemia is necessary for the development of diabetic nephropathy, it is not sufficient; some patients escape nephropathy despite relatively poor diabetic control. Other factors must therefore play a role in the pathogenesis, perhaps proteinuria itself – excessive tubular protein uptake induces release of vasoactive and inflammatory cytokines, mononuclear cell infiltration and renal injury. Hypertension is also critical to the development of diabetic nephropathy. Transmitted pressure to the glomerular capillaries causes mechanical stretch of glomerular component cells and stimulation of matrix components such as collagen. Hyperglycaemia and mechanical stretch both activate intracellular signalling pathways, which stimulate growth factors [e.g. transforming growth factor-β_1 (TGF-β_1) and vascular endothelial growth factor (VEGF)] and cytokines, *via* the important intracellular mediator, protein kinase C (PKC; see Chapter 14).

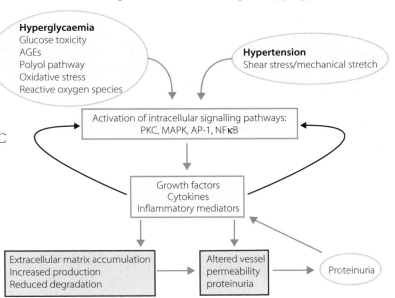

FIGURE 16.13
Mechanisms involved in the pathogenesis of diabetic nephropathy. AGE, advanced glycation end-product; AP-1, activator protein-1 transcription factor; MAPK, mitogen-activated protein kinases; NFκB, nuclear factor-κB; PKC, protein kinase C.

159

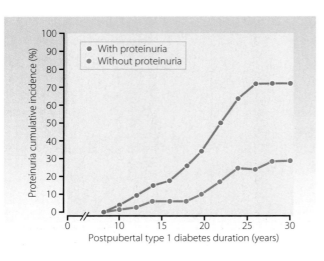

Diabetic nephropathy tends to cluster in families; it is more likely in type 1 diabetic siblings of a diabetic patient who has proteinuria than in siblings of a patient without proteinuria. The genetic component of individual susceptibility to diabetic nephropathy remains unexplained, although there is evidence that a familial predisposition to hypertension may contribute.

FIGURE 16.14
The cumulative incidence of persistent proteinuria in type 1 diabetic siblings of probands with type 1 diabetes, with proteinuria or without proteinuria.

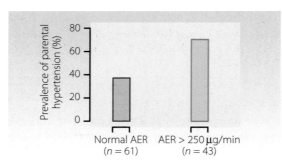

The risk of developing nephropathy is increased three-fold if at least one parent has hypertension. Several candidate genes display polymorphisms associated with diabetic nephropathy (e.g. angiotensin-converting enzyme, angiotensinogen and angiotensin 2 type 1 receptor), but their individual contributions appear to be small (and remain controversial). Most likely, there is a complex interaction between the effects of several genes and multiple environmental factors.

FIGURE 16.15
The prevalence of hypertension is increased in parents of those with proteinuria, which suggests that genetic predisposition may influence the development of nephropathy. AER, albumin excretion rate.

Management in those patients with microalbuminuria consists of normalization of blood pressure (aiming for a BP <130/75 mmHg) and correction of cardiovascular risk factors. Their special effects on renal haemodynamics and greater anti-proteinuric effects mean that ACE inhibitors are the therapy of first choice. They may also have cardioprotective benefits. However, combination therapy is often required for the control of blood pressure (see Chapter 19). Some physicians now use low-dose ACE inhibitors in microalbuminuric subjects who are normotensive.

FIGURE 16.16
Management of microalbuminuria.

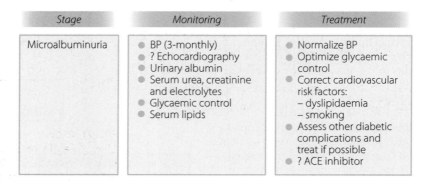

Stage	Monitoring	Treatment
Microalbuminuria	• BP (3-monthly) • ? Echocardiography • Urinary albumin • Serum urea, creatinine and electrolytes • Glycaemic control • Serum lipids	• Normalize BP • Optimize glycaemic control • Correct cardiovascular risk factors: – dyslipidaemia – smoking • Assess other diabetic complications and treat if possible • ? ACE inhibitor

HANDBOOK OF DIABETES 3RD EDITION

In patients with overt proteinuria, renal function must be monitored to estimate prognosis and determine the effects of intervention. A 24-hour urine collection quantifies protein excretion, and urine should be examined microscopically and cultured to exclude infection. Ultrasound scanning can indicate renal artery stenosis. Serum creatinine does not increase until the GFR has fallen by 50–70%, so ideally GFR should be measured in the early stages by isotopic methods. Plots of inverse creatinine [i.e. 1000 ÷ (creatinine), in µmol/L] show a linear decline when the serum creatinine exceeds 200 µmol/L.

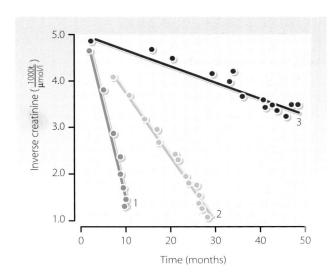

FIGURE 16.17
Inverse serum creatinine declines linearly with time, at a fixed rate for each individual patient (fastest for patient 1 and slowest for patient 3).

Early effective blood pressure control (<140/80 mmHg) is again important in overt proteinuria, and typically reduces the rate of decline in GFR from about 12 to <5 mL/min/year. Metformin and most sulphonylureas are cleared by the kidney and accumulate with uraemia, which causes hypoglycaemia (sulphonylureas) and toxic effects. Metformin should be withdrawn when the serum creatinine is >150 µmol/L, because of the risk of lactic acidosis. Transfer to insulin is therefore recommended when the serum creatinine exceeds 200 µmol/L. As renal failure progresses, insulin requirements fall because of reduced renal clearance and degradation of insulin. There is limited evidence that reducing protein intake to 0.7–1.0 g/kg body weight per day slows the decline in GFR in type 1 diabetes. Aspirin should also be considered because of the high risk of cardiovascular events in these patients.

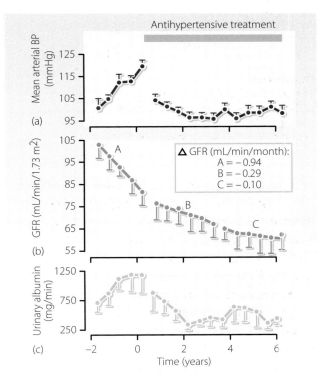

FIGURE 16.18
Effects of antihypertensive treatment on (a) mean arterial blood pressure; (b) GFR; and (c) urinary albumin excretion in type 1 diabetes patients with nephropathy. Rates of decline in both GFR and albumin excretion were significantly reduced.

161

Referral to a nephrology unit is generally recommended when the serum creatinine approaches 200–250 µmol/L. Renal replacement therapy consists of haemodialysis, continuous ambulatory peritoneal dialysis (CAPD) and renal transplant. Renal transplant is the treatment of choice for patients under the age of 60 years and should be considered when the serum creatinine reaches 500–800 µmol/L. Simultaneous renal–pancreas transplant may be an option. Older patients have a particularly poor prognosis because of cardiovascular disease, and are generally offered dialysis rather than transplantation. Full cardiovascular investigation is mandatory before acceptance for transplantation. The 5-year patient survival (>80% for grafts from live-related donors) in diabetes is now as good as that in the non-diabetic population.

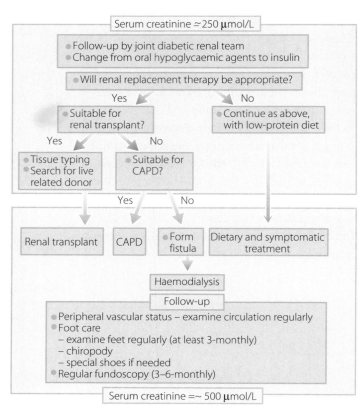

FIGURE 16.19
Management of renal failure in diabetes.

Haemodialysis poses special problems for the diabetic patient, as vascular access may be technically difficult because of atherosclerosis and medial calcification. Arteriovenous fistulae may fail prematurely. Satisfactory and stable metabolic control may be difficult to achieve, while hypotension during dialysis may make it impossible to remove sufficient fluid. The alternative of CAPD is inexpensive and does not require vascular access; extracellular fluid and blood pressure are stable, and it is more suitable for elderly patients and those with heart failure or autonomic neuropathy. Insulin may be administered intraperitoneally during CAPD.

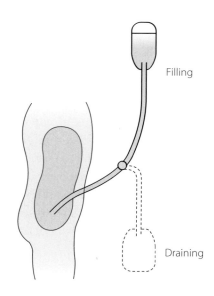

FIGURE 16.20
Continuous ambulatory peritoneal dialysis (CAPD). Dialysis fluid is instilled by gravity into the peritoneal cavity and drained after a dwell period of several hours.

HANDBOOK OF DIABETES 3RD EDITION

Various clinical syndromes of diabetic neuropathy are recognized. Nerve damage can be classified into an acute and reversible 'hyperglycaemic neuropathy', and other persistent neuropathies, such as distal symmetrical and focal and multifocal neuropathies.

Hyperglycaemic neuropathy occurs in patients whose diabetes has been controlled poorly for weeks or months, when uncomfortable sensory symptoms appear in the lower legs, and clear when control improves. Nerve conduction velocity is slowed. The mechanism is unknown.

A. Acute reversible

Hyperglycaemic neuropathy

B. Persistent

1. Symmetrical

   Distal symmetrical neuropathy (chronic sensory and autonomic polyneuropathy)

   Acute painful neuropathy

2. Focal and multifocal

   Pressure palsies

   Mononeuropathies (diabetic amyotrophy)

FIGURE 17.1
A classification of diabetic nephropathies.

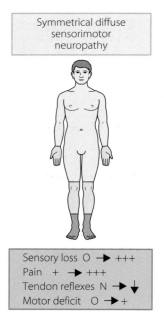

Sensory loss O ➜ +++
Pain + ➜ +++
Tendon reflexes N ➜ ↓
Motor deficit O ➜ +

The most common neuropathy is *distal symmetrical neuropathy* (or 'chronic sensory and autonomic polyneuropathy') – the 'classic' diabetic peripheral neuropathy. This results from the distal dying back of axons that begins in the longest nerves; thus, the feet are affected first, in a stocking distribution, and there may be later progressive involvement of the upper limbs. Sensory loss is most evident; autonomic involvement (see below) is usual, although it is mostly symptomless.

FIGURE 17.2
Clinical pattern of distal symmetrical neuropathies.

Symptoms in distal symmetrical neuropathy

• Asymptomatic in some

• Numbness

• Altered sensation
  – paraesthesiae
  – allodynia

• Pain

Sensory symptoms include numbness, paraesthesiae, allodynia (contact sensitivity) and pain (burning or like an electric shock). Distal symmetrical neuropathy may also be symptomless, but the feet are at risk because sensory deficits can lead to damage.

FIGURE 17.3
Symptoms in distal symmetrical neuropathy.

HANDBOOK OF DIABETES 3RD EDITION

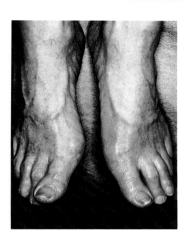

These patients have warm, dry feet, because of autonomic involvement, which results in dilated arteriovenous shunts and absent sweating. The most important complications are:

- Foot ulceration.
- Neuropathic oedema, caused by increased blood flow in the foot, which has sympathetic innervation damage.
- Charcot arthropathy, with chronic destruction, deformity and inflammation of the joints and bone. There is reduced bone density, possibly because of increased blood flow (see Chapter 21).

FIGURE 17.4
Increased blood flow (distended veins) on the dorsum of the foot of a diabetic patient with painful peripheral neuropathy.

Examination may reveal distal symmetrical loss of vibration sense (tuning fork), touch (cotton wool or 10 g nylon monofilament), pinprick, joint position sense and temperature. However, the objective signs may be less impressive than are suggested by the patient's symptoms. Formal measurements of vibration sense with a biothesiometer and nerve conduction studies are not generally required in clinical practice.

Signs in distal symmetrical neuropathy

- None

- Loss of
  – vibration sense
  – pin prick
  – touch
  – temperature
  – joint position sense

- Wasting and weakness rare

- Complications (ulcer, oedema, Charcot arthropathy)

FIGURE 17.5
Signs in distal symmetrical neuropathy.

Acute painful diabetic neuropathy is a distinct syndrome of symmetrical neuropathy, characterized by acute and extremely severe pain, burning or lancinating in nature, and with contact sensitivity. This often follows rapid weight loss, usually in the context of poor glycaemic control (Fig. 17.6). It may occur with newly diagnosed diabetes, with the acute metabolic disruption of ketoacidosis or with an eating disorder. The symptoms usually remit over 12–24 months, generally in parallel with improvements in weight.

FIGURE 17.6
Relationship between painful neuropathic symptoms and changes in body weight. Initiation of treatment with insulin is indicated by the arrow, treatment before then having been with an oral hypoglycaemic agent. A sudden loss of over 27 kg in weight was accompanied by the development of a mild and then a severe neuropathy. Restoration of body weight was associated with improvement and then disappearance of the neuropathy.

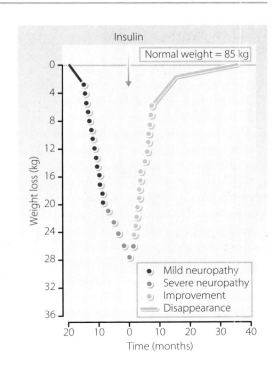

Pressure palsies comprise focal lesions of peripheral nerves that occur at sites of entrapment or compression. Diabetic nerves are thought to be more susceptible to mechanical injury. The most common is the carpal tunnel syndrome (median nerve compression), in which paraesthesiae and sometimes numbness occur in the fingers and hands. Discomfort can radiate into the forearm. Examination can show wasting and weakness of the thenar muscles, with loss of sensation over the lateral three-and-a-half fingers. The diagnosis can be confirmed by nerve conduction studies. Most patients respond to surgical decompression.

Pressure palsies

Ulnar

Lateral
popliteal

Median

Sensory loss	+ → +++
Pain	+ → ++
Tendon reflexes	N
Motor deficit	+ → +++

FIGURE 17.7
Clinical pattern of pressure palsies.

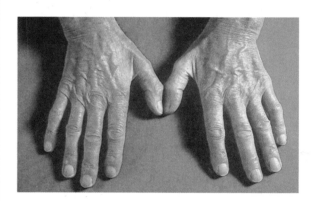

Ulnar nerve compression at the elbow causes numbness and weakness of the fourth and fifth fingers and wasting of the interossei muscles. Lateral popliteal nerve compression can cause foot drop.

FIGURE 17.8
Generalized wasting of the interossei (and hypothenar eminence) caused by bilateral ulnar nerve palsies in a diabetic patient.

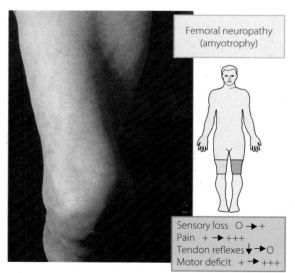

Femoral neuropathy
(amyotrophy)

Sensory loss	O → +
Pain	+ → +++
Tendon reflexes	↓ → O
Motor deficit	+ → +++

FIGURE 17.9
Diabetic amyotrophy, showing marked quadriceps wasting, and clinical pattern (inset).

In mononeuropathies, single nerves or their roots are affected and, in contrast to distal symmetrical neuropathy, these conditions are of rapid onset and reversible, which suggests an acute, possibly vasculitic or inflammatory origin rather than chronic metabolic disturbance. The best known is femoral neuropathy or diabetic amyotrophy. There is multifocal involvement of the lumbosacral roots, plexus and femoral nerve. Typically, the patient is over 50 years of age, with continuous thigh pain, wasting and weakness of the quadriceps, and sometimes weight loss. The knee jerk reflex is lost. Climbing the stairs or getting out of bed may be difficult. One or both thighs may be affected. Recovery is usually spontaneous, but may take many months.

HANDBOOK OF DIABETES 3RD EDITION

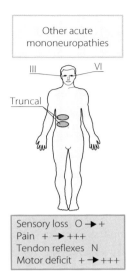

Other acute
mononeuropathies

III   VI

Truncal

Sensory loss O ➔ +
Pain + ➔ +++
Tendon reflexes N
Motor deficit + ➔ +++

Other mononeuropathies include cranial nerve palsies that affect the third or sixth nerves (causing sudden-onset diplopia). The cause is thought to be a localized infarct that involves brainstem nuclei or nerve roots. Older people are mainly affected. Truncal (thoraco-abdominal) neuropathy causes localized bulging of the abdominal wall, either unilaterally or bilaterally. It may be accompanied by burning or a lancinating girdle-like pain, similar to shingles. It is rare.

FIGURE 17.10
Clinical patterns of cranial and truncal mononeuropathies.

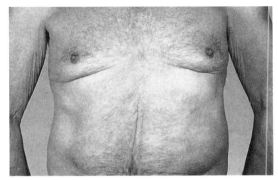

FIGURE 17.11
Bulging of the left lower abdominal wall caused by truncal radiculopathy.

In patients with long-standing diabetes, numerous abnormalities can be demonstrated in organs that receive an autonomic innervation. Often, autonomic abnormalities are found in those with distal sensory neuropathies. Symptoms are unusual, occurring mostly in those with poorly controlled type 1 diabetes. Common manifestations are gustatory sweating over the face (induced by eating cheese or other foods), postural hypotension (systolic blood pressure fall >30 mmHg on standing), blunting of physiological heart-rate variations, diarrhoea and impotence. Gastroparesis (delayed gastric emptying and vomiting) and bladder dysfunction are rare.

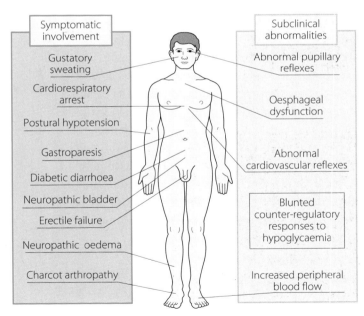

Symptomatic involvement
- Gustatory sweating
- Cardiorespiratory arrest
- Postural hypotension
- Gastroparesis
- Diabetic diarrhoea
- Neuropathic bladder
- Erectile failure
- Neuropathic oedema
- Charcot arthropathy

Subclinical abnormalities
- Abnormal pupillary reflexes
- Oesphageal dysfunction
- Abnormal cardiovascular reflexes
- Blunted counter-regulatory responses to hypoglycaemia
- Increased peripheral blood flow

FIGURE 17.12
Clinical and subclinical features of diabetic autonomic neuropathy.

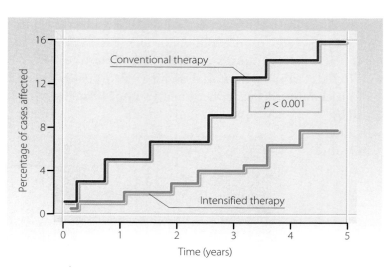

FIGURE 17.13
Effects of intensified insulin therapy and strict glycaemic control on the incidence of neuropathy in type 1 diabetic patients (DCCT).

Management of diabetic neuropathy begins with explanation and empathy, the exclusion of other causes of neuropathy (e.g. alcoholism, vitamin B12 deficiency and uraemia), and then the institution of tight glycaemic control. Both the DCCT and UKPDS trials showed that strict glycaemic control can decrease the risk of developing neuropathy, as judged by objective measures such as nerve conduction velocity. However, the main complaint of patients with neuropathy is pain, and there is as yet little evidence that improving diabetic control influences the intensity of neuropathic pain.

Simple analgesics such as paracetamol (acetaminophen), aspirin and codeine phosphate only rarely have an effect on diabetic neuropathic pain. Burning pain can be controlled by tricyclic antidepressants such as amitriptyline and imipramine given at night. Capsaicin (derived from hot peppers) is also useful, applied twice daily to the skin as cream; it releases the peptide neurotransmitter, substance P, from the pain-fibre nerve endings, leading to depletion of the nerves and insensitivity for some hours. Allodynia may respond to a bed cradle or a protective film (OpSite, Smith and Nephew Ltd) applied to the skin. Electric shock-like or shooting pains may be treated with anticonvulsants (carbamazepine, gabapentin, phenytoin, valproate) or the orally active form of lignocaine (lidocaine), mexiletine. Restless legs are best managed by the benzodiazepine, clonazepam. Cramps are generally helped by quinine sulphate at night.

FIGURE 17.14
Approach to the management of painful diabetic neuropathy.

General measures

Improve glycaemic control
Exclude or treat other contributory factors
- Alcohol excess
- Vitamin B12 deficiency
- Uraemia
Explanation, empathy and reassurance

Choose drugs according to the patient's dominant symptoms

Burning pain
1 Tricyclic drugs
- Imipramine
- Amitriptyline ± fluphenazine
2 Capsaicin

Lancinating pain
1 Anticonvulsants
- Gabapentin
- Carbamazepine
- Phenytoin or valproate
2 Tricyclic agents
3 Capsaicin

Other symptoms
Contact discomfort (allodynia)
- Plastic film (OpSite) on legs

Restless legs
- Clonazepam

Painful cramps
- Quinine sulphate

BLOOD LIPID ABNORMALITIES 18

Lipid abnormalities are common in type 2 diabetic patients, even in those who have reasonable glycaemic control. The characteristic disturbance in type 2 diabetes is called 'diabetic dyslipidaemia', which also occurs in the metabolic or insulin resistance syndrome ('syndrome X') and impaired glucose tolerance. It consists of elevated serum total and VLDL (very low-density lipoprotein) triglyceride, low HDL (high-density lipoprotein) and essentially normal total and LDL (low-density lipoprotein) cholesterol concentrations. Overproduction of triglyceride-rich VLDL by the liver and impaired triglyceride clearance by endothelial lipoprotein lipase are contributory factors. The distribution of LDL subfractions is altered, however, with a predomination of small, dense LDL particles (the 'type B' pattern), which are more susceptible to oxidation and are highly atherogenic. These abnormalities of dyslipidaemia are not reversed completely by tight metabolic control.

Diabetic dyslipidaemia
↑ Triglyceride
↑ VLDL triglyceride
↑ Small dense LDL
↓ HDL-cholesterol

FIGURE 18.1
Diabetic dyslipidaemia.

Dyslipidaemia associated with the metabolic syndrome and type 2 diabetes is also accompanied by a prothrombotic state (increased fibrinogen and plasminogen activator inhibitor-1, PAI-1) and by proinflammatory changes [increased acute-phase proteins such as C-reactive protein (CRP) and their cytokine mediators such as interleukin-6 and tumour necrosis factor α; see Chapter 7]. These abnormalities substantially increase the risk of cardiovascular disease. Dyslipidaemia is an acute-phase response, characteristic of inflammation.

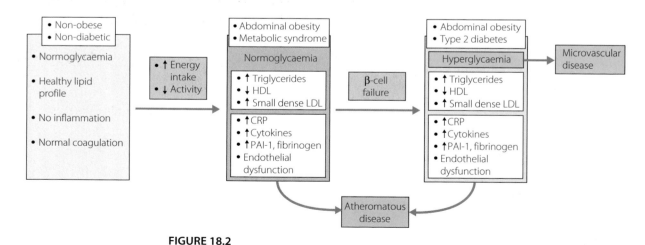

FIGURE 18.2
Cluster of atherogenic metabolic abnormalities that result from abdominal obesity and are shared with patients with type 2 diabetes. Even before type 2 diabetes supervenes, the abdominally obese patient with the metabolic syndrome carries a high risk of coronary heart disease. CRP, C-reactive protein; HDL, high-density lipoprotein; LDL, low-density lipoprotein; PAI-1, plasminogen activator inhibitor-1.

In non-obese, well-controlled type 1 diabetes, serum lipid and lipoprotein concentrations are similar to those in non-diabetic people. In poorly controlled type 1 diabetes, hypertriglyceridaemia can occur because insulin deficiency causes increased lipolysis, overproduction of non-esterified fatty acids and VLDL, and decreased activity of endothelial lipoprotein lipase, which reduces clearance of triglyceride-containing VLDL and chylomicrons. Very high triglyceride levels (>20 mmol/L) can occur in poorly controlled or newly presenting type 1 diabetic patients, often in association with ketoacidosis. Complications include eruptive xanthomas in the skin, acute pancreatitis and lipaemia retinalis (a milky appearance of the retinal vessels seen on ophthalmoscopy). The main determinants of hyperlipidaemia in type 1 diabetes are age, obesity, poor glycaemic control and nephropathy.

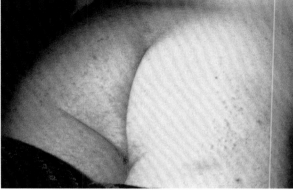

FIGURE 18.3
Eruptive xanthoma.

Total serum cholesterol and triglyceride and HDL cholesterol concentration should be measured routinely in diabetic patients, preferably in fasting blood samples. LDL cholesterol can be calculated (i.e. without direct measurement of LDL by ultracentrifugation) from the Friedewald equation (all concentrations in mmol/L; triglyceride should be less than 5 mmol/L):

$$LDL\ chol = [total\ chol] - [HDL\ chol] - \frac{[total\ triglyceride]}{2.2}$$

(note that this formula may be less accurate in diabetic than in normal subjects).

Fasting lipid profile as part of annual review

↓

Lipid profile 'acceptable'
- Cholesterol < 5.2 mmol/L
- Triglyceride < 2.3 mmol/L
- HDL cholesterol > 1.1 mmol/L

↓

Repeat annually

FIGURE 18.4
Routine lipid measurements.

Investigation of hyperlipidaemia in diabetes should exclude other secondary hyperlipdaemias, notably those that can coexist with diabetes, such as hypothyroidism, drugs (e.g. alcohol, some antihypertensive agents) and renal disease. Primary hyperlipidaemia must also be remembered; severe hypertriglyceridaemia or hypercholesterolaemia in diabetic patients often results from an underlying primary disorder, exacerbated by poorly controlled diabetes.

Other medical disorders	Main lipid abnormalities
Alcohol abuse	↑ Triglyceride, ↑ HDL
Therapeutic drugs (diuretics, oral contraceptives, retinoids, corticosteroids, anabolic steroids, progestogens related to testosterone)	↑ Triglyceride and/or cholesterol, ↓ HDL
Hypothyroidism	↑ Cholesterol
Chronic renal failure	↑ Triglyceride
Nephrotic syndrome	↑ Cholesterol, ± ↑ triglyceride
Cholestasis	↑ Cholesterol
Bulimia	↑ Triglyceride
Anorexia nervosa	↑ Cholesterol
Pregnancy	↑ Triglyceride

Dyslipidaemias induced by antihypertensive drugs

	Total cholesterol	Total triglyceride	LDL cholesterol	HDL cholesterol
Calcium antagonists				
Vasodilators	N	N	N	N
ACE inhibitors				
α-blockers	N↓	N↓	N↓	N↑
Diuretics	↑	↑	↑	N
β-blockers				
• Non-selective	N	↑	N	↓
• Intrinsic sympathomimetic activity	N	↑	N	N↑
• Vasodilator properties	N	N	N	N

FIGURE 18.5
Secondary hyperlipidaemia. N, no effect; ↑, ↓, reduced, increased levels.

Management of diabetic dyslipidaemia begins with lifestyle modification – dietary restriction for the obese, with increased physical exercise, aiming to promote weight loss. A low-fat, lipid-lowering diet may be beneficial. General measures include improving glycaemic and blood pressure control and cessation of smoking. Other identified causes of hyperlipidaemia should be treated.

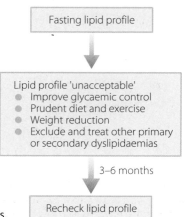

Fasting lipid profile

Lipid profile 'unacceptable'
● Improve glycaemic control
● Prudent diet and exercise
● Weight reduction
● Exclude and treat other primary or secondary dyslipidaemias

3–6 months

Recheck lipid profile

FIGURE 18.6
Treatment of hyperlipidaemia: initial measures.

HANDBOOK OF DIABETES 3RD EDITION

If hyperlipidaemia persists after these measures, lipid-lowering drugs should be considered. In general, the thresholds for the active management of hyperlipidaemia by drugs have fallen in recent years. In deciding on the need for drug therapy, it may be helpful to stratify patients according to the risk associated with the serum lipid levels.

Risk	LDL-cholesterol (mg/dL)	(mmol/L)	HDL-cholesterol (mg/dL)	(mmol/L)	Triglycerides (mg/dL)	(mmol/L)
High	≥ 130	≥ 3.4	< 35	<0.9	≥ 400	≥ 4.6
Borderline	100–129	2.6–3.3	35–45	0.9–1.2	200–399	2.3-4.5
Low	< 100	<2.6	> 45	>1.2	< 200	<2.3

FIGURE 18.7
Category of risk based on lipoprotein levels in adults.

Statins (HMG-CoA reductase inhibitors) are the drugs of choice for lowering cholesterol. Examples include simvastatin, pravastatin, fluvastatin, rosuvastatin and atorvastatin). They work by inhibiting an early step in cholesterol synthesis, reducing hepatic cholesterol production by up to 40%, which secondarily upregulates LDL receptor synthesis and thus promotes the removal of LDL cholesterol and VLDL remnant particles from the blood. LDL cholesterol falls by up to 40% and triglyceride by about 20%. Some statins (e.g. atorvastatin) are more effective at lowering triglycerides. The drugs are generally safe and well tolerated. Myositis is a rare adverse effect, but is more frequent when statins are used with fibrates, nicotinic acid or ciclosporin.

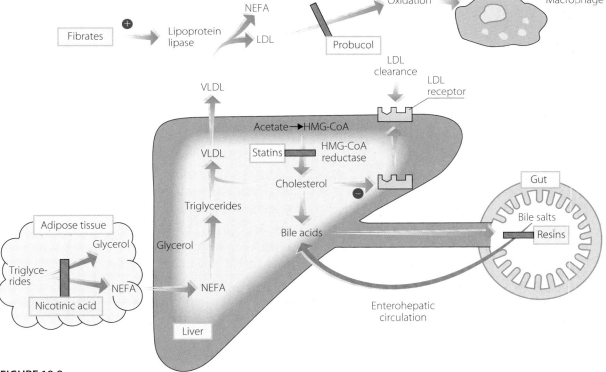

FIGURE 18.8
Modes of action of lipid-lowering drugs. Resins block the enterohepatic circulation of the bile acids by binding bile acids in the gut. This leads to increased bile acid synthesis and requirement for cholesterol in the liver. Nicotinic acid blocks lipolysis in adipose tissue, which lowers non-esterified fatty acids (NEFA) and thus hepatic triglyceride and VLDL. Probucol blocks LDL oxidation and hence uptake by macrophages. Statins inhibit HMG-CoA reductase, which reduces cellular cholesterol, up-regulating LDL receptor synthesis and LDL removal from the blood.

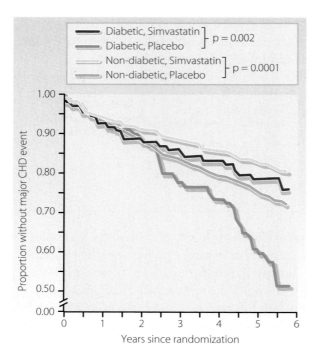

FIGURE 18.9
'4S' trial of the effect of simvastatin vs placebo on CHD incidence in type 2 diabetes and non-diabetic subjects.

Several clinical trials have shown a reduction in cardiovascular events with statin treatment in diabetic subjects, though varying in magnitude. In the Scandinavian Simvastatin Survival Study (the '4S Trial'), simvastatin-treated patients with diabetes showed reductions in major coronary heart disease (CHD) events and revascularization procedures of 42% and 48%, respectively. A reduction in CHD events (including death) was also found in the CARE (Cholesterol and Recurrent Events) trial of pravastatin (25%) and in the Long-term Intervention with Pravastatin in Ischaemic Disease (LIPID) study (19%).

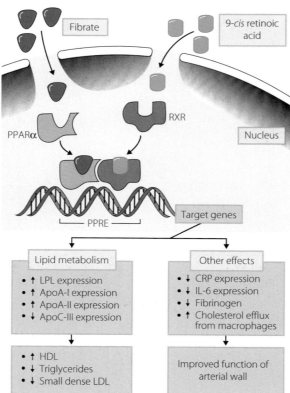

FIGURE 18.10
The mechanism of action of fibrates. PPRE, peroxisome proliferator response element; LPL, lipoprotein lipase; CRP, C-reactive protein; IL-6, interleukin-6; RXR, retinoid X receptor.

Fibric acid derivatives (bezafibrate, fenofibrate, gemfibrozil, ciprofibrate) are useful for the treatment of hypertriglyceridaemia and mixed hyperlipidaemia, lowering serum triglyceride and increasing HDL cholesterol concentrations. Their mechanism of action involves binding to the nuclear receptor, peroxisome proliferator-activated receptor α (PPARα). This forms a complex with another nuclear receptor, retinoid X receptor (RXR), and interacts with the response elements of several genes that control lipoprotein metabolism (e.g. increasing the expression of the lipoprotein lipase gene and thus increasing triglyceride breakdown). Some other non-lipid risk factors may also be lowered by fibrates, including PAI-1, fibrinogen and CRP. Several trials show that fibrates reduce CHD events in diabetes and they appear particularly beneficial in patients with low HDL, central obesity and other features of the metabolic syndrome.

Other lipid-lowering agents, such as bile acid sequestrants (e.g. cholestyramine), probucol and nicotinic acid and its derivatives (e.g. acipimox), are currently little used in diabetes.

Hypertension is up to twice as common in diabetes as in the general population, and affects some 10–30% of type 1 and 30–50% of type 2 diabetic patients. It is also present in about 20–40% of people with impaired glucose tolerance. However, there are some racial differences in the prevalence of hypertension, with a lower frequency in native Americans (Pima Indians) and Mexican Americans. Hypertension is rather broadly defined by the World Health Organization (WHO) and the International Society for Hypertension (ISH), but because diabetic people with hypertension are at risk of macrovascular and microvascular complications below these WHO and ISH thresholds, the treatment target range (desirable blood pressure) is generally considered lower in diabetes – <130–140/85 mmHg, and lower (<125/80) in those with nephropathy.

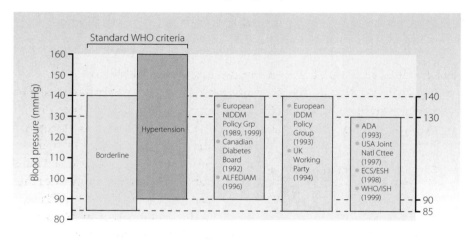

FIGURE 19.1
Blood pressure treatment targets suggested for diabetic subjects, compared with the World Health Organization/International Society for Hypertension definition of hypertension and borderline hypertension.

In type 2 diabetes, hypertension is associated with insulin resistance and other features of the metabolic syndrome (central obesity, dyslipidaemia and macrovascular disease). Other links between diabetes and hypertension include nephropathy, diabetogenic antihypertensive drugs (e.g. some diuretics and β-blockers), drugs that cause both diabetes and glucose intolerance (e.g. glucocorticoids) and endocrine disorders that cause both diabetes and hypertension (e.g. Cushing's syndrome, acromegaly, Conn's syndrome and phaeochromocytoma). Essential hypertension, which is common in the general population, can also coexist with diabetes (accounting for perhaps 10% of cases in diabetes).

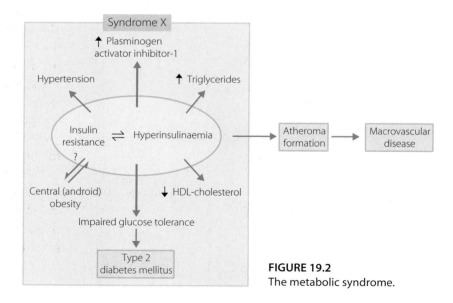

FIGURE 19.2
The metabolic syndrome.

Hypertension associated with type 2 diabetes mellitus ('syndrome X')

Hypertension associated with nephropathy in type 1 diabetes mellitus

Coincidental hypertension in diabetic patients
- Essential hypertension
- Isolated systolic hypertension
- Renal scarring, e.g. from recurrent pyelonephritis

Diabetogenic antihypertensive drugs
- Potassium-losing diuretics (chlorthalidone, high-dose thiazides)
- β-blockers (high dose)
- Combined diuretics and β-blockers

Drugs causing both hypertension and glucose intolerance
- Glucocorticoids
- Combined oral contraceptive pills

Endocrine disorders causing hypertension and glucose intolerance
- Acromegaly
- Cushing's syndrome
- Conn's syndrome
- Phaeochromocytoma

FIGURE 19.3
Associations between hypertension and diabetes.

There are several ways in which insulin resistance and/or hyperinsulinaemia could lead to hypertension. One is blunting of the vasodilator effect of insulin (an action mediated by the release of nitric oxide from endothelium). On the other hand, insulin has other actions that raise blood pressure, which could be accentuated by the hyperinsulinaemia that accompanies insulin resistance. For example, insulin stimulates sodium and water absorption at the distal renal tubule. Insulin also stimulates the cell membrane Na^+-K^+ ATPase, which could raise intracellular Na^+ and Ca^+ in vascular smooth muscle and thereby enhance contractility and peripheral resistance. Through its effects on the central nervous system, insulin may stimulate sympathetic outflow, and insulin may also stimulate the proliferation of vascular smooth muscle cells. Several components of the augmented cytokine-induced, acute-phase (inflammatory) response associated with type 2 diabetes (see Chapter 7) may cause hypertension, including cytokine stimulation of ACTH and glucocorticoid secretion, and activation of the sympathetic nervous system.

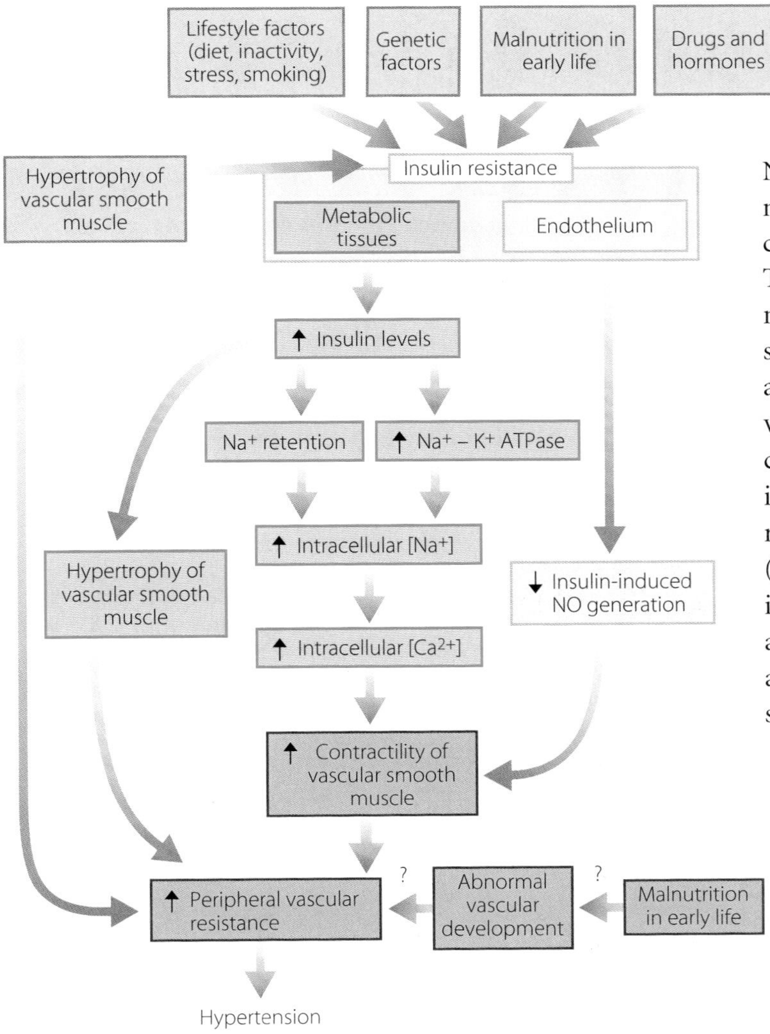

FIGURE 19.4
Possible mechanisms of hypertension in conditions of insulin resistance. NO, nitric oxide.

In type 1 diabetes, hypertension is most obviously associated with diabetic nephropathy (see Chapter 16). Blood pressure begins to rise when the albumin excretion rate enters the microalbuminuric range (>30 mg/24 h). The association of hypertension and diabetic nephropathy may be partly genetically determined.

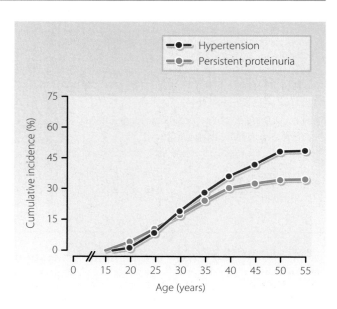

FIGURE 19.5
Hypertension rises in parallel with proteinuria in type 1 diabetes patients of various ages.

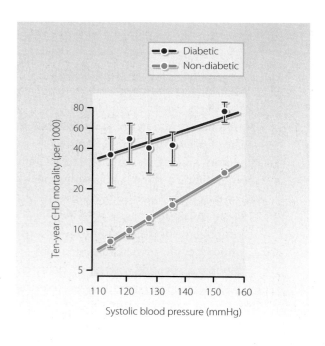

Control of hypertension in diabetes is important because hypertension worsens both macrovascular and microvascular complications. The effect of blood pressure on the risk of fatal coronary heart disease is 2–5 times greater in diabetic than in non-diabetic people. Hypertension also accentuates the deleterious effects of diabetes on left ventricular mass and function.

FIGURE 19.6
Synergistic effects of diabetes and hypertension on deaths from coronary heart disease (CHD). Data from 342 815 non-diabetic and 5163 diabetic subjects aged 35–57 years, free from myocardial infarction at entry.

The deleterious effect of hypertension on micro- and macrovascular complications was demonstrated clearly in the United Kingdom Prospective Diabetes Study (UKPDS, reported 1998), in which 1148 type 2 diabetic patients with hypertension were allocated to either tight control or less tight control of blood pressure (mean BP over 9 years 144/82 vs 154/87 mmHg). Not only was there a large reduction in the risk of strokes in the tight blood pressure group (44%), but also in that of microvascular endpoints (37%), including retinopathy and microalbuminuria.

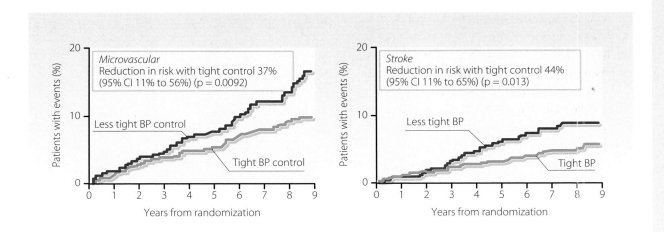

FIGURE 19.7
Kaplan–Meier plots of proportions of patients who developed microvascular endpoints (mostly retinal photocoagulation), and fatal and non-fatal strokes during tight or less tight BP control (UKPDS).

Initial investigations in hypertensive patients must exclude rare causes of secondary hypertension, such as Cushing's and Conn's syndromes and phaeochromocytoma. Damage to the kidney (microalbuminuria or proteinuria, urine microscopy, serum urea, creatinine and electrolytes) and cardiovascular system (electrocardiogram or echocardiography, chest radiograph for left ventricular hypertrophy) must be assessed. Specialist investigations may be needed to identify renal artery stenosis, which may affect up to 20% of older type 2 diabetic patients. Other cardiovascular risk factors should be identified (hyperlipidaemia, poor glycaemic control, smoking, family history).

Investigations	Questions to be answered
History	Is hypertension significant?
Cardiovascular symptoms	Does hypertension have
Previous urinary disease	an underlying cause?
Smoking and alcohol use	• Renal
Medication	• Endocrine
Family history of hypertension	• Drug-induced
or cardiovascular disease	Has hypertension caused
	tissue damage?
Examination	• Left-ventricular
Blood pressure erect and supine	hypertrophy
Left-ventricular hypertrophy	• Ischaemic heart
Cardiac failure	disease
Peripheral pulses (including renal	• Cardiac failure
bruits and radio-femoral delay)	• Peripheral vascular
Fundal changes of hypertension	disease
Evidence of underlying endocrine	• Renal impairment
or renal disease	• Fundal changes
	Are other cardiovascular
Electrocardiogram	risk factors present?
Left-ventricular hypertrophy	• Smoking
Ischaemic changes	• Hyperlipidaemia
Rhythm	• Poor glycaemic control
	• Positive family history
Chest radiograph	of cardiovascular disease
Cardiac shadow size	
Left-ventricular failure	
Echocardiography	
Left-ventricular hypertrophy	
Dyskinesia related to ischaemia	
Blood tests	
Urea, creatinine, electrolytes	
Fasting lipids	

FIGURE 19.8
Investigation of the diabetic patient with hypertension.

179

General measures for the treatment of hypertension include weight reduction in the obese, a low fat/low sodium diet, increased physical exercise, institution of strict glycaemic control, reduced alcohol intake, cessation of smoking and management of hyperlipidaemia. Few patients respond to lifestyle modification alone, and most will require antihypertensive drug treatment. Patients with severe hypertension (diastolic >110 mmHg) or with signs of hypertensive damage generally need drugs from the outset. Numerous drugs are available to lower blood pressure, and it is usual to start with monotherapy. There are a variety of relative indications and contraindications for each class of antihypertensive. About two-thirds of diabetic patients eventually require combinations of two or more agents to control blood pressure.

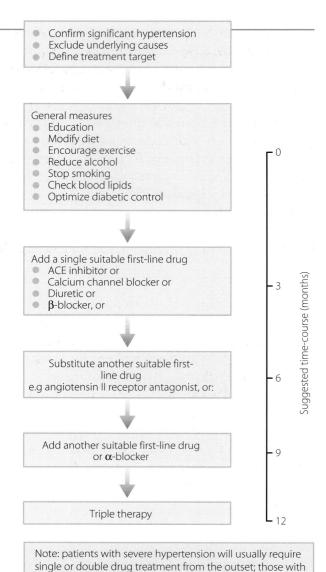

FIGURE 19.9
Suggested management scheme for diabetic patients with hypertension. Drug treatment should be started as shown if hypertension remains uncontrolled after 3 months of general measures.

Note: patients with severe hypertension will usually require single or double drug treatment from the outset; those with lesser degrees of hypertension frequently respond to general measures alone

FIGURE 19.10
Properties of ACE inhibitors.

Group	Examples	Relative indications	Relative contraindications	Precautions
ACE inhibitors	Captopril Enalapril Lisinopril Perindopril Fosinopril Trandolapril Cilazapril Ramipril Quinapril	Cardiac failure Proteinuria	Renal artery stenosis Renal impairment	First-dose hypotension (use small starting dose at night) Monitor renal function Monitor plasma potassium (risk of hyperkalaemia)

ACE inhibitors are popular first-line agents because they are effective in lowering blood pressure and also delay the progression of diabetic retinopathy, reduce microalbuminuria (even in those without hypertension) and slow the progression to renal failure. Their antiproteinuric effect may result from relaxation of the efferent glomerular arterioles, thus reducing intraglomerular hypertension. They have no adverse effects on lipid profiles or glycaemic control, but dry cough (in 10–15% of patients) and potassium retention are recognized side-effects. ACE inhibitors should not be taken with potassium-sparing diuretics (spironolactone and amiloride). Renal failure may occasionally be precipitated in those with renal artery stenosis. Exaggerated postural hypotension may occur with the first dose, especially in those overtreated with diuretics or with autonomic neuropathy; a low starting dose, given at bedtime, is therefore sensible. ACE inhibitors are also indicated in cardiac failure, in combination with low-dosage diuretics. Ramipril has been shown to reduce by 25% the risk of a combined endpoint of myocardial infarction, stroke or cardiovascular disease death in type 2 diabetic subjects with microalbuminuria (the MICRO-HOPE study). ACE inhibitors are less effective in Afro-Caribbean patients

Angiotensin II receptor antagonists are a new class of anti-hypertensive drugs that block the action of angiotensin at its AT_1 receptor. Losartan was the first to be introduced, and several others (e.g. irbesartan, valsartan and candesartan) are now available. They are metabolically neutral and do not cause cough; at the moment, the clearest indication for these drugs is for patients in whom cough prevents the use of ACE inhibitors. Angiotensin II receptor antagonists, like ACE inhibitors, slow the progression of nephropathy in diabetes.

Angiotensin II receptor antagonists

- Losartan
- Valsartan
- Irbesartan
- Candesartan
- Telmisartan

FIGURE 19.11
Angiotensin II receptor antagonists.

Calcium channel blockers are vasodilators that usually have no adverse metabolic actions. Mild ankle oedema is a side-effect, while postural hypotension in those with autonomic neuropathy is exacerbated. As a result of the vasodilator actions, they are useful in hypertensive patients with angina, but should not be used in those with heart failure because of an additional action of reduction in cardiac contractility – most potently with verapamil. The vasodilator properties may also be beneficial in those with peripheral vascular disease. The special combination of verapamil and β-blockers (especially with digoxin) must be avoided because of the risk of conduction block and asystole.

Group	Examples	Relative indications	Relative contraindications	Precautions
Calcium-channel blockers	Nifedipine Amlodipine Diltiazem Verapamil Isradipine	Angina Arrhythmias	Significant cardiac failure Treatment with digoxin + β-blocker (verapamil)	Autonomic neuropathy (aggravate postural hypotension)

FIGURE 19.12
Properties of calcium-channel blockers.

A low dose of the thiazide diuretic, bendrofluazide (2.5 or even 1.25 mg/day) effectively lowers blood pressure in many patients; the risk of worsened glycaemic control and aggravated dyslipidaemia seen with thiazides is minimal at these low doses. Impotence and the precipitation of hyperosmolar non-ketotic coma are possible side-effects. If renal function is impaired (serum creatinine >150 μmol/L), thiazides are ineffective and loop diuretics such as frusemide (furosemide) are recommended. Low-dose thiazide diuretics are often favoured in elderly type 2 diabetic patients because of the proved efficacy in reducing stroke and mortality in the elderly hypertensive person.

Group	Examples	Relative indications	Relative contraindications	Precautions
Diuretics	Bendrofluazide Hydrochlorothiazide Indapamide Frusemide	Cardiac failure Renal failure (frusemide)	Hyperosmolar coma Impotence Gout Hyperlipidaemia	Give with potassium supplements or ACE inhibitors Monitor blood potassium Check blood glucose and lipids

FIGURE 19.13 Properties of diuretics.

β-adrenoreceptor blockers act mainly by reducing cardiac output and are often used in those with angina or previous myocardial infraction. Atenolol and metoprolol are cardioselective. Propranolol and timolol are non-cardioselective and also act on bronchiolar smooth muscle to cause bronchospasm; β-blockers are contraindicated in patients with asthma. Like diuretics, they may aggravate hyperglycaemia, dyslipidaemia and impotence, but the effects can be minimized by using low doses combined with other agents. β-blockers interfere with the counter-regulatory effects of catecholamines released during hypoglycaemia, thereby blunting tachycardia and tremor, and delaying glycaemic recovery. However, this rarely causes problems in clinical practice, particularly if cardioselective agents are used. β-blockers are generally contraindicated in heart block and severe peripheral vascular disease. Metoprolol and carvedilol may be indicated in patients who also have heart failure. Other problems with β-blockers (especially non-cardioselective) are vivid dreams and cold hands and feet. Like ACE inhibitors, β-blockers are often less effective in Afro-Caribbean subjects.

Group	Examples	Relative indications	Relative contraindications	Precautions
β-blockers	Atenolol Metoprolol Propranolol Pindolol Carvedilol* Bisopropril Nebivolol Acebutolol	Angina Previous myocardial infarction	Cardiac failure Heart block Peripheral vascular disease Impotence Asthma, chronic airflow obstruction Hyperlipidaemia	Warn about loss of hypoglycaemic awareness Monitor blood glucose and lipids

FIGURE 19.14 Properties of β-blockers.

HANDBOOK OF DIABETES 3RD EDITION

Other antihypertensive agents useful in diabetes include α_1-blockers such as doxazosin. This improves dyslipidaemia and insulin sensitivity as well as blood pressure. It is normally well tolerated; side-effects include nasal congestion and postural hypotension. It is particularly used in combination therapy, especially in type 2 diabetic patients with dyslipidaemia.

- α_1-blockers
  e.g. doxazosin, prazosin

- Hydralazine

FIGURE 19.15
Other antihypertensives used in diabetes.

Combination therapy is needed in most diabetic patients to achieve satisfactory blood pressure control. To minimize side-effects, it is often better to use low-dose drug combinations than to increase the dose of single agents. Combinations that have proved safe and effective in low-to-moderate dose include ACE inhibitor plus calcium channel blocker, ACE inhibitor plus diuretic, selective β-blocker plus calcium channel blocker and β-blocker plus α_1-blocker.

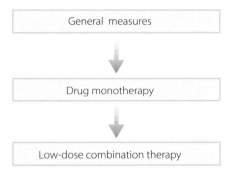

FIGURE 19.16
Strategy for the management of hypertension.

MACROVASCULAR DISEASE IN DIABETES

20

The frequencies of coronary heart disease, stroke and peripheral vascular disease are all about 2–4 times higher in either type 1 or type 2 diabetes compared with the general population. Cardiovascular disease (CVD) is the most common cause (about 75%) of death in type 2 diabetes. Both genders are affected; notably, women lose their normal premenstrual protection against CVD. The co-existence of diabetes and nephropathy (proteinuria) increases the risk of CVD mortality still further. Certain ethnic groups are particularly susceptible to CVD in association with diabetes (e.g. South Asians in the UK and blacks in the USA), while others are relatively protected (native Americans, such as the Pima Indians, and Hispanic whites in the USA).

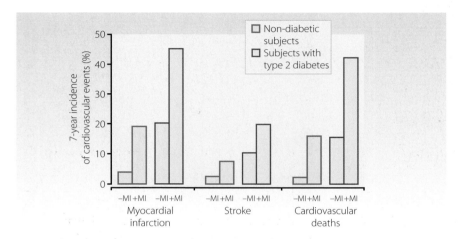

FIGURE 20.1
Cardiovascular risk in event-free diabetic patients is comparable to that in non-diabetic subjects who have already had a myocardial infarct. The 7-year incidence of myocardial infarction, stroke and cardiovascular death in diabetic and non-diabetic subjects categorized by past history of vascular disease. + MI, previous infarct; –MI, no previous infarct.

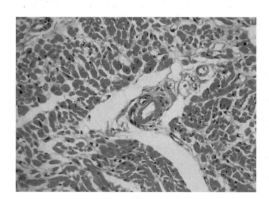

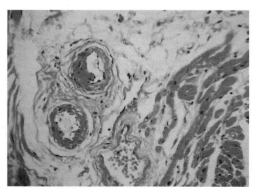

The pathology of atheroma in diabetes is identical to that in non-diabetic people. Crucially, though, it develops earlier and faster and is more extensive, as it involves distal vessels in both the coronary and peripheral circulation. The coronary lesions are more prone to plaque ulceration and instability, which predisposes to thrombus formation, occlusion and thus unstable angina or myocardial infarction. The main structural changes in diabetes are thickening of the arterial wall intima (which can be detected in young adults and precedes obvious atheroma) and 'hyaline' change in the media, caused by the degeneration of arterial wall proteins, like collagen, and the uptake of glycated plasma proteins.

FIGURE 20.2
Arteriolar changes in diabetes, in the myocardium of a woman who died from renal failure caused by diabetic nephropathy. There is thickening of the basement membrane and periodic acid–Schiff (PAS)-positive staining material in the artery wall. The changes in this patient are likely to have involved hypertension as well as diabetes. Haematoxylin and eosin stain.

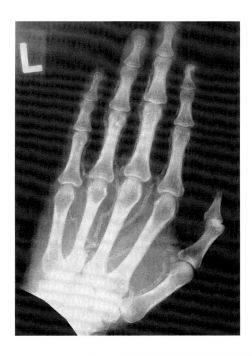

The small and medium arteries and arterioles are damaged further by microvascular disease in the vasa vasorum, which reduces blood supply and makes the media prone to calcification – 'Mönckeberg's medial sclerosis' – often clearly seen in the digital arteries of diabetic patients with nephropathy and/or neuropathy.

FIGURE 20.3
Medial calcification of the digital arteries in a diabetic patient with severe arterial disease and nephropathy.

Major functional abnormalities in the endothelium in diabetes include increased endothelial adhesiveness 'which favours macrophage and platelet attachment', impaired vasodilatation [e.g. from decreased nitric oxide (NO) production], enhanced haemostasis and increased permeability (which allows plasma lipoproteins to enter the arterial media).

FIGURE 20.4
Main effects of diabetes on the walls of arteries and arterioles. AGE, advanced glycation end-product; NO, nitric oxide.

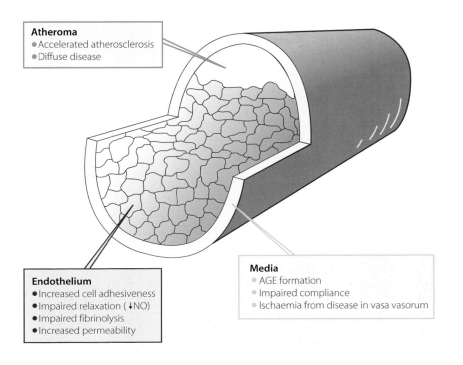

Atheroma
- Accelerated atherosclerosis
- Diffuse disease

Endothelium
- Increased cell adhesiveness
- Impaired relaxation (↓NO)
- Impaired fibrinolysis
- Increased permeability

Media
- AGE formation
- Impaired compliance
- Ischaemia from disease in vasa vasorum

The major cardiovascular risk factors in the non-diabetic population – smoking, hypertension and hyperlipidaemia – also operate in diabetes, but the risks are enhanced in the presence of diabetes. This was demonstrated strikingly in the Multiple Risk Factor Intervention Trial (MRFIT).

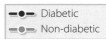

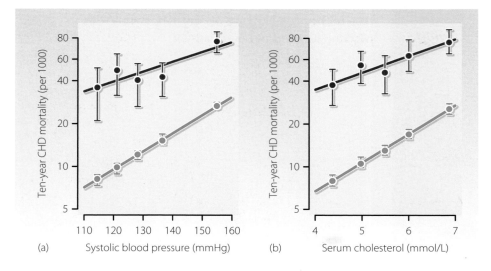

FIGURE 20.5
Effects of (a) systolic blood pressure and (b) serum cholesterol concentration on 10-year mortality from coronary heart disease (CHD) in 342 815 non-diabetic and 5163 diabetic subjects aged 35–57 years who initially had not suffered myocardial infarction.

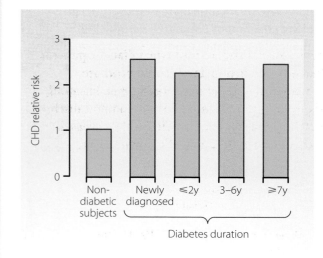

The risk associated with diabetes itself is not explained fully. Cardiovascular risk rises as blood glucose increases in the subdiabetic range; but, unlike microvascular disease, there is a relatively weak relationship in established diabetes between macrovascular disease and either duration of diabetes or the level of glycaemic control. In both the Diabetes Control and Complications Trial (DCCT) in type 1 diabetes and the UK Prospective Diabetes Study (UKPDS) in type 2 diabetes, improved glycaemic control had no significant effect on cardiovascular outcomes.

FIGURE 20.6
Relative risk of coronary heart disease (CHD) in type 2 diabetes is not obviously related to the duration of diabetes.

Nevertheless, there are several mechanisms by which hyperglycaemia could contribute to macrovascular disease. Advanced glycation end products (AGEs, see Chapter 14) cross-link vessel-wall proteins, which causes thickening and leakage and traps plasma proteins in the subintimal layers. AGEs also generate toxic reactive oxygen species that quench the vasodilator NO and so favour vasoconstriction. Many of the effects of AGEs are mediated by their interaction with specific receptors (RAGEs) on the endothelium, smooth muscle cells, monocytes and macrophages, including upregulation of procoagulant (e.g. PAI-1) and adhesive (e.g. VCAM-1) proteins, and attraction of monocytes that form the foam cells which initiate the atheromatous plaque.

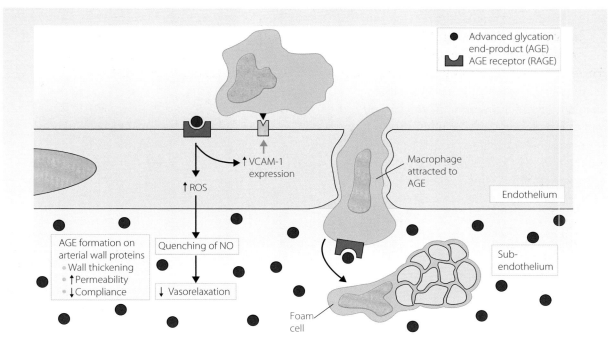

FIGURE 20.7
Some effects of advanced glycation end-products (AGEs) on the arterial wall. NO, nitric oxide; ROS, reactive oxygen species; VCAM-1, vascular cell adhesion molecule-1.

Hyperinsulinaemia is present in many type 2 diabetic patients and in most type 1 diabetic patients who receive insulin injections. The suggestion that elevated insulin levels could promote atherosclerosis in diabetes has been debated for many years and remains a theoretical risk. Harmful, potentially atherogenic and/or hypertensive effects of insulin include stimulation of smooth muscle cell proliferation and migration, enhanced sympathetic outflow, stimulation of cholesterol synthesis in macrophages and smooth muscle cells, and retention of sodium and water by the renal tubule.

As mentioned above, atheromatous risk factors tend to cluster with insulin resistance in syndrome X, or the metabolic syndrome (see Chapters 7, 18 and 19). The syndrome's features include type 2 diabetes or impaired glucose tolerance, dyslipidaemia, hypertension and central obesity. Other components of the metabolic syndrome are generally thought to be elevated plasma uric acid and procoagulant factors, such as fibrinogen and PAI-1.

FIGURE 20.8
The 'insulin resistance syndrome' (metabolic syndrome X).

189

Diabetes may also damage the myocardium directly, in the absence of coronary heart disease. Histologically, there is interstitial fibrosis and microvascular changes (basement membrane thickening and microaneurysms). The main subclinical features are abnormalities of left ventricular contractility demonstrated on echocardiography, which generally correlate with the duration of diabetes and the extent of microvascular complications. More severe left ventricular dysfunction leads to heart failure. Arrhythmias are associated with left ventricular hypertrophy and may be responsible for some cases of sudden, unexplained death, especially in young type 1 diabetic people.

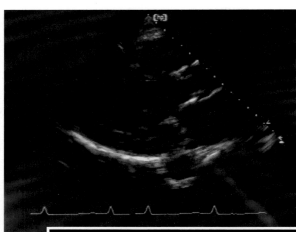
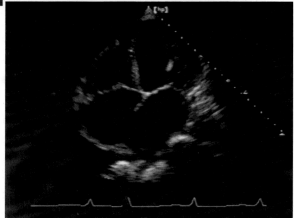

FIGURE 20.9
Echocardiogram in a diabetic patient with severe congestive cardiac failure. (a) Long-axis, two-dimensional image in systole, showing dilated left atrium (51 mm) and left ventricle (55 mm). (b) Four-chamber, two-dimensional image in systole, showing biatrial and biventricular enlargement. There was global hypokinesia; dilation of the valve rings caused functional mitral and tricuspid regurgitation, despite normal valves.

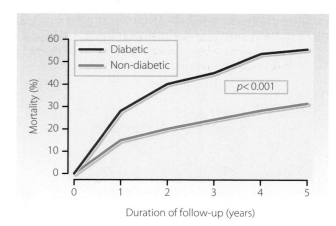

FIGURE 20.10
Five-year mortality among diabetic and non-diabetic patients during follow-up after myocardial infarction.

The presentation of ischaemic heart disease in diabetes includes angina, myocardial infarction and heart failure, as it does in the non-diabetic population. However, angina and myocardial infarction may be relatively painless ('silent') in diabetes, especially in older people (perhaps because of neuropathic damage to the autonomic nerves that serve the myocardium); symptoms such as malaise, sweating, nausea, dyspnoea and syncope may be ignored or confused with hypoglycaemia. Both immediate and long-term mortality from myocardial infarction are increased in diabetes, largely through the increased risk of heart failure in diabetes (because of diabetic cardiomyopathy, superimposed hypertension and loss of functioning myocardium after coronary occlusion).

HANDBOOK OF DIABETES 3RD EDITION

Transient ischaemic attacks and stroke are also common in diabetes, and mortality and disability after a stroke are greater in diabetes, compared with non-diabetic people. The cause remains uncertain.

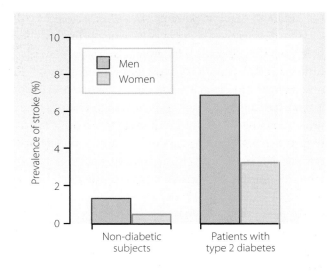

FIGURE 20.11
Age-adjusted prevalence of previous stroke in type 2 diabetes subjects compared with control subjects (45–64 years of age).

Arterial disease in the legs typically presents with intermittent claudication (i.e. calf pain on walking). Buttock pain may occur if the iliac vessels are affected and may be associated with erectile failure (the Leriche syndrome). Decreasing claudication distance or rest pain indicate critical ischaemia. People with diabetes have an approximately 16-fold higher risk of leg amputation than non-diabetic people (see Chapter 21). About 20% of those with peripheral vascular disease die within 2 years of the onset of symptoms, mostly from myocardial infarction.

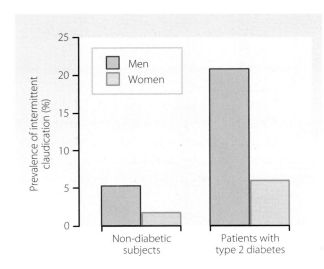

FIGURE 20.12
Age-adjusted prevalence of intermittent claudication in type 2 diabetic subjects compared to control subjects (45–64 years of age).

Angina in diabetic patients should be managed conventionally; cardioselective β-blockers may be particularly useful. Aspirin should also be given and other risk factors managed aggressively. If symptoms worsen, early consideration should be given to coronary angiography and revascularization (see below). Acute coronary syndromes without myocardial infarction (unstable angina) have a high risk of progressing to myocardial infarction in diabetes and require intensive treatment with low molecular weight heparin, a β-blocker and either the platelet inhibitor, clopidogrel, or an inhibitor of platelet glycoprotein IIb/IIIa, such as tirofiban or eptifibatide. Urgent coronary revascularization is indicated if medical measures fail.

Primary prevention	Acute event	Secondary prevention
Healthy eating	*Acute coronary syndrome*	As for primary, with:
Exercise	Low-molecular weight heparin	• Aspirin
Non-smoking	Clopidogrel	• β-blocker, and/or ACE inhibitor
Lose weight if obese	[GpIIb/IIIa inhibitor]	• Clopidogrel (if ACS)
BP < 135/85 mmHg	Revascularization	• Risk-factor reduction
Normal HbA$_{1c}$		• Consider revascularization
Aspirin	*Acute myocardial infarct*	
[Statin]	Thrombolysis	
[Fibrate]	Intravenous insulin/glucose	
[ACE inhibitor]	β-blocker	
	ACE inhibitor	

FIGURE 20.13
Primary prevention of myocardial infarction, management of acute coronary syndrome and myocardial infarction, and secondary preventative measures.

Acute myocardial infarction should be treated with immediate thrombolysis (e.g. with streptokinase or recombinant tPA, even in the presence of retinopathy), as well as aspirin and a cardioselective β-blocker. If the patient is not already receiving an ACE inhibitor, one should be started (unless there is hypotension and renal impairment), so as to reduce the risk of heart failure.

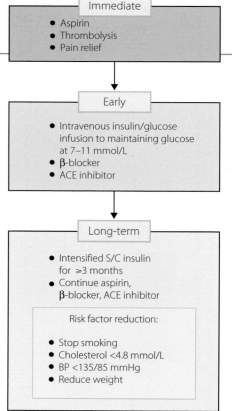

FIGURE 20.14
Management of uncomplicated myocardial infarction in diabetic patients. ACE, angiotensin-converting enzyme; S/C, subcutaneous.

Blood glucose should be controlled tightly, according to the 'DIGAMI' protocol. This derives from the Diabetes Mellitus Insulin Glucose Infusion in Acute Myocardial Infarction study, which showed a 30% reduction in mortality in diabetic patients treated with insulin soon after infarction, compared with conventional management. This involves an insulin–glucose solution infused intravenously to maintain blood glucose levels of 7–11 mmol/L for at least 24 hours, followed by intensive subcutaneous insulin treatment for at least 3 months. It is unclear at the moment whether the benefits in the DIGAMI study result from the acute effects of insulin or longer-term influences.

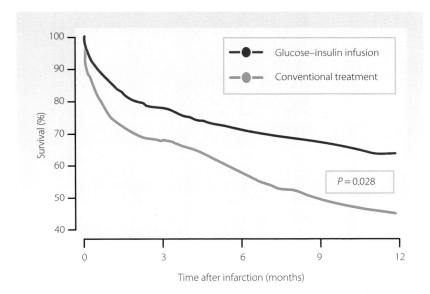

FIGURE 20.15
Intravenous insulin–glucose infusion to achieve tight glycaemic control after myocardial infarction reduces mortality in patients found to be hyperglycaemic on admission.

FIGURE 20.16
Glucose–insulin infusion protocol to achieve tight glycaemic control after acute myocardial infarction.

Infusion mixture

Add 80 units soluble insulin to 500 mL 5% glucose

Infuse initially at 30 mL/h

Measure blood glucose every 1–2 h

Titrate infusion rate:

Blood glucose (mmol/L)	Adjustment
> 15.0	Give 8 units soluble insulin as IV bolus
	Increase infusion rate by 6 mL/h
11.0–14.9	Increase infusion rate by 3 mL/h
7.0–10.9	Maintain current rate
4.0–6.9	Decrease infusion rate by 6 mL/h
< 4.0	Stop infusion until glucose > 7 mmol/L
	Give 20 mL 30% glucose IV if symptomatic hypoglycaemia
	Restart infusion with rate decreased by 6 mL/h

Coronary revascularization relieves symptoms as effectively in diabetes as in non-diabetic people, but long-term survival is lower. It is technically more difficult in diabetes because of the typically diffuse and distal pattern of coronary atheroma. The preferred procedure for accessible, larger vessels is probably percutaneous transluminal coronary angioplasty with stenting and probably a platelet inhibitor. Coronary artery bypass grafting (CABG) is generally reserved for difficult or multiple occlusions and for restenosis after angioplasty.

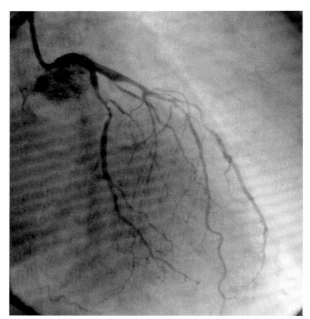

FIGURE 20.17
Diffuse coronary artery disease in a 49-year-old woman with type 1 diabetes mellitus. The coronary angiogram shows widespread involvement of the mid-zones of both the left anterior descending and circumflex coronary arteries. She underwent successful coronary artery bypass grafting.

HANDBOOK OF DIABETES 3RD EDITION

Foot problems are a major demand on diabetes care, the most common lesions being foot ulcers, with or without infection, and gangrene. In westernized countries, about 7% of diabetic patients have foot ulcers at any one time. This is the most common reason for hospitalization and the most expensive complication of diabetes (20% of total costs). Charcot arthropathy and neuropathic oedema are rare. The leg amputation rate among diabetic patients is over 15 times that in non-diabetic subjects.

The diabetic foot

- Foot ulcers
- Gangrene
- Charcot arthropathy
- Neuropathic oedema

FIGURE 21.1
The diabetic foot.

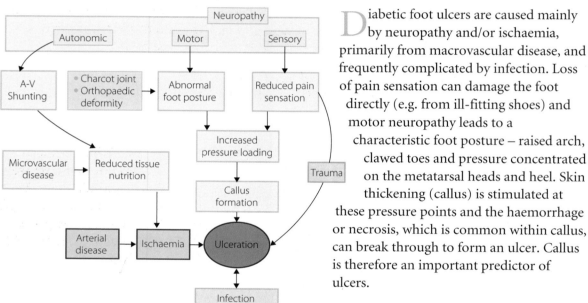

FIGURE 21.2
Aetiology of foot ulceration in diabetic patients.

Diabetic foot ulcers are caused mainly by neuropathy and/or ischaemia, primarily from macrovascular disease, and frequently complicated by infection. Loss of pain sensation can damage the foot directly (e.g. from ill-fitting shoes) and motor neuropathy leads to a characteristic foot posture – raised arch, clawed toes and pressure concentrated on the metatarsal heads and heel. Skin thickening (callus) is stimulated at these pressure points and the haemorrhage or necrosis, which is common within callus, can break through to form an ulcer. Callus is therefore an important predictor of ulcers.

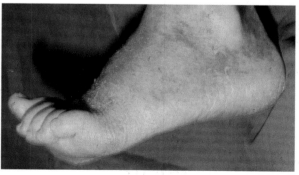

FIGURE 21.3
Neuropathic foot, showing clawed toes, dry skin and prominent veins.

Autonomic nerve damage leads to reduced sweating, which leads to dry and cracked skin and so allows the entry and spread of infection. Damage to the sympathetic innervation of the foot leads to arteriovenous shunting and distended veins. This bypasses the capillary bed in affected areas and may compromise nutrition and oxygen supply. Microvascular disease may also interfere with nutritive blood supply to the foot tissues.

HANDBOOK OF DIABETES 3RD EDITION

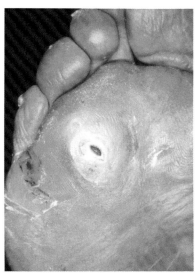

FIGURE 21.4
Typical neuropathic ulcer. Note the surrounding callus.

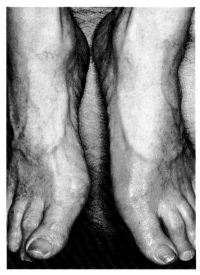

FIGURE 21.5
Distended veins on the dorsum of the foot of a diabetic patient with painful peripheral neuropathy.

Neuropathic ulcers represent about one-half of foot lesions, and typically occur in high-pressure areas, such as over the metatarsal heads on the plantar surface of the foot or on the heal or toes. They often have a 'punched-out' appearance, with surrounding callus. The foot may be warm from the shunting of cutaneous blood flow. Signs of neuropathy are present (e.g. reduced pin-prick, touch and temperature sensation).

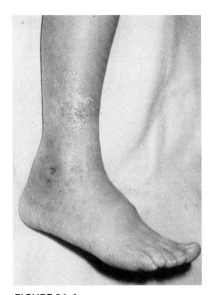

FIGURE 21.6
Neuroischaemic ulcer over the lateral malleolus. Note the hairless, thin skin of the leg.

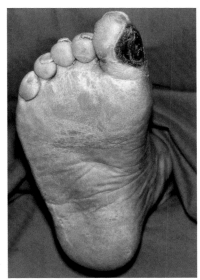

FIGURE 21.7
Neuroischaemic damage caused by tightly fitting shoes.

Neuroischaemic ulcers (10–30% of ulcers) are often ragged edged, on the margins of the feet and painful. The foot is cool and pulseless, with loss of hair and thin skin on the legs.

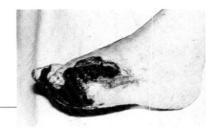

FIGURE 21.8
Gangrene localized to the forefoot in a neuroischaemic foot.

Predominantly ischaemic lesions result in gangrene that is localized to a specific area of the foot or to the entire foot, depending on the level of arterial occlusion.

Infection usually enters the foot through cracked skin or ulcers and can spread to deep tissues, sometimes with the risk of osteomyelitis. Signs of infection include local erythema, crepitus (from gas, in infections with gas-forming organisms), and contact with bone on probing ulcers or sinuses (which generally indicates osteomyelitis). Systemic disturbance, such as fever and leukocytosis, are usually absent, unless septicaemia develops. With osteomyelitis, plain radiography may reveal gas formation or bone erosion. Additional imaging may be needed, using ^{99m}Tc bone scanning, labelled white cell scanning (specific for local infection) or computer tomography (CT) with magnetic resonance (MR) imaging, to distinguish from other causes of bone destruction, such as Charcot arthropathy.

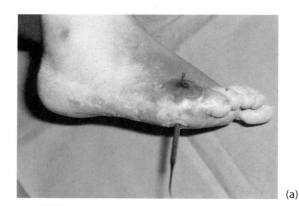

(a)

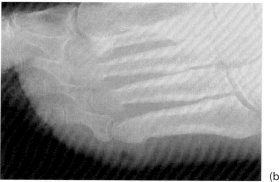

(b)

FIGURE 21.9
Osteomyelitis. Bone was contacted on probing the sinus penetrating the fifth metatarsal head (a). (b) Initial plain radiograph, showing early osteomyelitic changes and gas in the soft tissues, which is caused by air in the sinus.

Charcot arthropathy is a rare complication of severe neuropathy in long-standing diabetes. The initiating event may be an injury (perhaps unnoticed) that causes bone fracture. Repeated minor trauma in pain-insensitive feet and possibly enhanced blood flow caused by sympathetic denervation may predispose to reduced bone density. Excessive osteoclast activity leads to bone resorption, coalescence and remodelling that can result in joint destruction and gross deformity. Over months, the patient may notice the foot changing shape or the sensation or sound of the bones crunching on walking. In the later stages, a large effusion may surround disrupted joints and bone fragments – the 'bag of bones' appearance on an X-ray (Fig. 21.11).

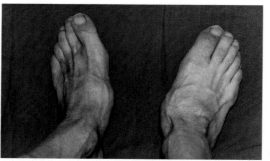

(a)

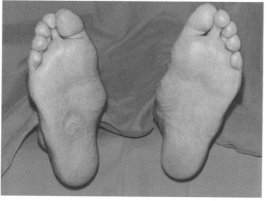

(b)

FIGURE 21.10
Bilateral Charcot neuroarthropathy in the cuneiform–metatarsal area that has resulted in characteristic deformity: (a) dorsal and (b) plantar views.

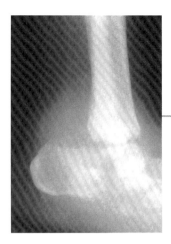

FIGURE 21.11
Charcot foot. Gross destruction of the ankle joint, with an effusion. The classic 'bag of bones' appearance.

All diabetic patients should have a regular screening examination of the feet, performed at least annually. Important points to note are:

- foot posture and shape, and callus at pressure points;
- site, appearance and infection of any ulcers present;
- evidence of neuropathy (including the warm skin and distended veins of autonomic damage);
- an assessment of vascular impairment (trophic changes, foot pulses).

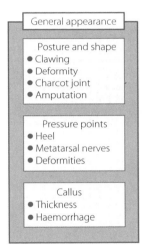
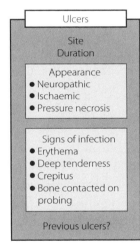
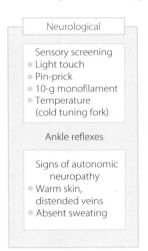
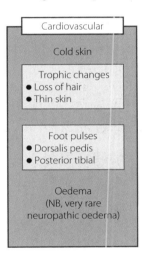

FIGURE 21.12
Checklist for examination of the foot in diabetic patients.

Treatment and prevention of foot ulcers requires specialized assistance from the chiropodist (podiatrist) and shoe-fitter (orthotist), who should work closely with the diabetes team and, when necessary, the orthopaedic and vascular surgeons. All patients must be educated about basic foot care and detection of abnormalities.

Target level of information to the needs and ability of the patient

Suggest 'dos' rather than 'don'ts' to encourage a positive approach

Do:
- Inspect feet daily
- Check shoes (inside and outside) before wearing them
- Have feet measured when buying shoes
- Buy lace-up shoes with plenty of room for toes
- Attend podiatrist regularly
- Keep feet away from heat (fires, radiators, hot water bottles) and check bath-water temperature before stepping in
- Wear protective footwear when indoors, or on the beach and avoid barefoot walking

Repeat the advice regularly

Also give advice to family members of the patient

FIGURE 21.13
General principles of foot-care education.

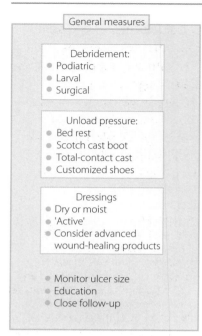

General measures

Debridement:
- Podiatric
- Larval
- Surgical

Unload pressure:
- Bed rest
- Scotch cast boot
- Total-contact cast
- Customized shoes

Dressings
- Dry or moist
- 'Active'
- Consider advanced wound-healing products

- Monitor ulcer size
- Education
- Close follow-up

FIGURE 21.14
General measures for the management of diabetic foot ulcers.

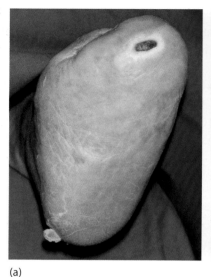
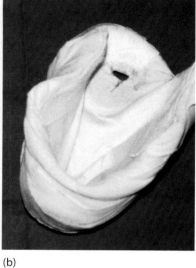

(a)   (b)

FIGURE 21.15
Neuropathic ulcer over the first and second metatarsal heads in a diabetic patient who (a) previously had the toes amputated for ulceration. (b) The foot was managed with a Scotchcast boot, with a hollow cut out under the ulcer area. Healing occurred within a few weeks.

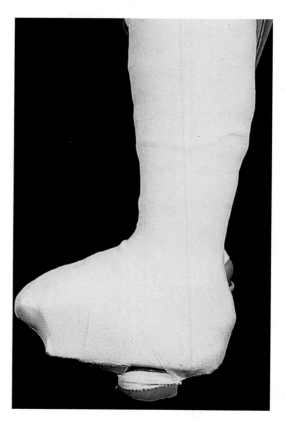

Management of neuropathic foot ulcers requires radical debridement (i.e. removal of callus and slough) and relief of pressure by bedrest with adequate heel support (which is difficult to enforce), off-loading foot supports, a total-contact cast or a removable Scotchcast boot. Radical debridement of neuroischaemic ulcers should be avoided because of poor wound healing in the foot with impaired circulation.

FIGURE 21.16
Total-contact plaster cast.

HANDBOOK OF DIABETES 3RD EDITION

The evidence base for the choice of ulcer dressing is not strong. Moist ulcer dressings that absorb exudate may promote granulation, but dry dressings are in common use. Newer treatments designed to accelerate wound healing are under evaluation, usually for the treatment of indolent plantar neuropathic ulcers that have failed to respond to conventional treatment. Dermograft® is a bioengineered human dermis that consists of neonatal fibroblasts cultured on a bioabsorbable mesh; the graft secretes matrix proteins and growth factors into the wound after application. Apligraf® is an alternative bilayered skin tissue. Becaplermin (Regranex®) is a gel that contains genetically engineered platelet-derived growth factor, which has been shown to accelerate healing of neuropathic ulcers. Autologous cultured keratinocytes grown in a laser-perforated hyaluronic acid membrane (Vivoderm Autograft System®) is also undergoing trial.

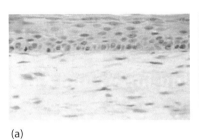
(a)

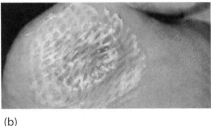
(b)

FIGURE 21.17
Bilayered skin tissue (Apligraf®). Keratinocytes and fibroblasts (prepared from neonatal human foreskin) are grown in culture as an upper 'epidermal' layer (keratinocytes) and a supporting 'dermal' layer of fibroblasts in a collagen matrix (a). The tissue is meshed before application to the ulcer (b).

Infection of diabetic foot ulcers can be superficial, or deep and potentially limb threatening, with abscesses and osteomyelitis. Antibiotic therapy should be targeted against identified organisms whenever possible, but this can be difficult to determine; pending identification, broad-spectrum antibiotics can be given. Superficial infection often responds to oral amoxicillin (co-amoxiclav) or clindamycin (which also penetrates bone and is useful for osteomyelitis). Deep infections and osteomyelitis can be treated with ampicillin and flucloxacillin, and metronidazole; or with ciprofloxacin and clindamycin (intravenously, then orally). Treatment may need to be continued for weeks.

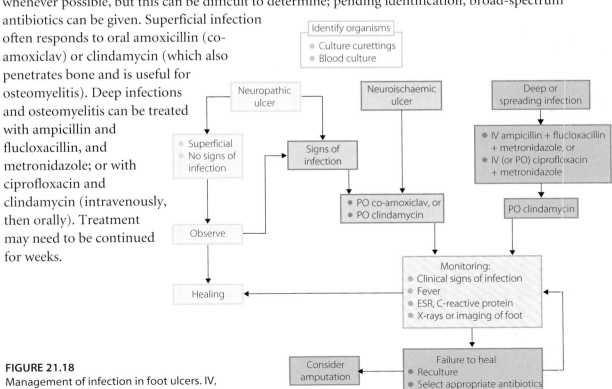

FIGURE 21.18
Management of infection in foot ulcers. IV, intravenous; PO, oral.

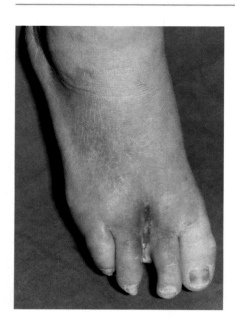

Full vascular assessment is mandatory for all patients who present with gangrene. Proximal reconstructive surgery and angioplasty are as effective as in the non-diabetic population. Gangrenous toes should be amputated, though localized areas of necrosis in toes with viable tissue borders can often be left to separate spontaneously ('autoamputation') and the residual wound treated as a neuroischaemic ulcer. Gangrene of the entire foot requires amputation, ideally below the knee; the extent of amputation can sometimes be reduced by prior reconstructive arterial surgery.

FIGURE 21.19
Surgical approaches to ischaemic lesions of the diabetic foot. This patient presented with a gangrenous third toe; arteriography revealed extensive stenosis in the superficial femoral artery. A femoral–popliteal bypass was performed successfully, and the gangrenous toe amputated. Healing followed in a few weeks, and the patient was fully mobile soon afterwards.

Erectile failure is the major sexual problem among diabetic men. It is more common than in the non-diabetic population and the frequency increases with age – it affects about 60% of diabetic men over the age of 60 years, with an overall prevalence of about 35–40%. The prevalence of erectile failure also tends to increase with diabetes duration and with co-existent cardiovascular disease, hypertension and smoking. Reduced libido and ejaculatory failure are other sexual problems that occur in diabetic men. Although attitudes to sexual dysfunction in diabetes have been transformed in recent years, the prevalence and impact are still probably underestimated.

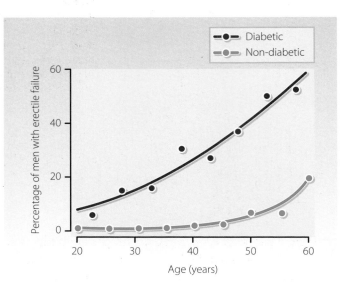

FIGURE 22.1
Prevalence of erectile failure in diabetic men.

Penile erection occurs as a result of engorgement of the erectile tissue following nitric oxide (NO)-mediated vascular smooth muscle relaxation in the corpus cavernosum (Fig. 22.2). NO is derived from both parasympathetic nerve endings and vascular endothelium. NO stimulates guanylate cyclase, which leads to increased production of the second messenger, cGMP, which induces smooth muscle relaxation (Fig. 22.3). Erectile dysfunction in diabetes mainly results from failure of NO-mediated relaxation, because of autonomic neuropathy and endothelial dysfunction.

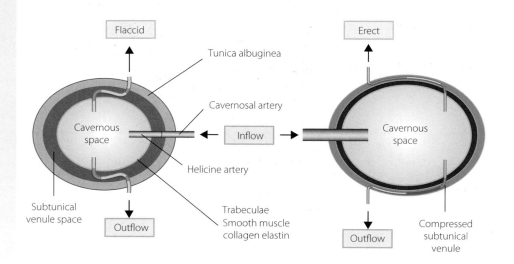

FIGURE 22.2
The corpus cavernosum. During tumescence, dilatation of the helicine and cavernosal arteries produces expansion of the cavernosal space and compression of the outflow venules against the rigid tunica albuginea.

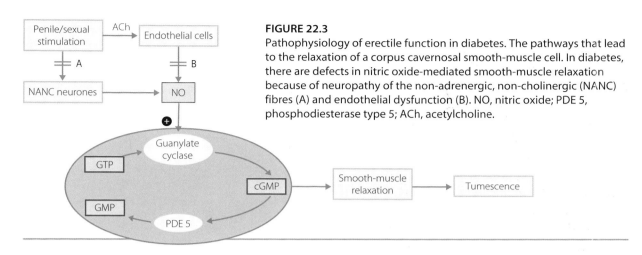

FIGURE 22.3
Pathophysiology of erectile function in diabetes. The pathways that lead to the relaxation of a corpus cavernosal smooth-muscle cell. In diabetes, there are defects in nitric oxide-mediated smooth-muscle relaxation because of neuropathy of the non-adrenergic, non-cholinergic (NANC) fibres (A) and endothelial dysfunction (B). NO, nitric oxide; PDE 5, phosphodiesterase type 5; ACh, acetylcholine.

Other factors that contribute to erectile failure in diabetes are arterial disease, drugs and a large number of psychological, neurological, endocrine, metabolic and other disorders that may co-exist with diabetes. The numerous drugs associated with erectile failure include alcohol, many anti-hypertensive agents (particularly β-blockers and thiazide diuretics) and anti-depressants. Reduced libido can be caused, at least in part, by the non-specific malaise of poor diabetic control, or the discomfort and anxiety associated with *Candida* balanitis (which is common with poor control).

Antihypertensives

Thiazide diuretics

β-blockers

Calcium-channel blockers

Angiotensin-converting enzyme (ACE) inhibitors

Central sympatholytics (methyldopa, clonidine)

Antidepressants

Tricyclics

Monoamine oxidase inhibitors

(NB: selective serotonin re-uptake inhibitors can cause ejaculatory problems)

Major tranquillizers

Phenothiazines

Haloperidol

Hormones

Luteinizing hormone-releasing hormone (goserelin, buserelin)

Oestrogens (diethylstilbestrol/stilboestrol)

Anti-androgens (cyproterone)

Miscellaneous

5α-reductase inhibitors (finasteride)

Statins (simvastatin, atorvastatin, pravastatin)

Cimetidine

Digoxin

Metoclopramide

Allopurinol

Ketoconazole

Non-steroidal anti-inflammatory agents

Fibrates

Drugs of 'abuse'/'social' drugs

Alcohol

Tobacco

Marijuana

Amphetamines

Anabolic steroids

Barbiturates

Opiates

FIGURE 22.4
Medications associated with erectile dysfunction.

Psychological disorders

Anxiety about sexual performance

Psychological trauma or abuse

Misconceptions

Sexual problems in the partner

Depression

Psychoses

Vascular disorders

Peripheral vascular disease

Hypertension

Venous leak

Pelvic trauma

Neurological disorders

Stroke

Multiple sclerosis

Spinal and pelvic trauma

Peripheral neuropathies

Endocrine and metabolic disorders

Diabetes

Hypogonadism

Hyperprolactinaemia

Hypopituitarism

Thyroid dysfunction

Hyperlipidaemia

Renal disease

Liver disease

Miscellaneous

Surgery and trauma

Smoking

Drug and alcohol abuse

Structural abnormalities of the penis

FIGURE 22.5
Conditions associated with erectile dysfunction.

A detailed history should be taken in men who complain of impotence, particularly to exclude related problems, such as premature ejaculation and loss of libido (which the patient may confuse with erectile failure), and to identify associated drugs and risk factors, such as smoking. General physical examination may give clues to the aetiology (e.g. hypogonadism), or indicate associated conditions such as balanitis, phimosis and Peyronie's disease, and cardiovascular disease.

FIGURE 22.6
Key features in the clinical history of diabetic erectile dysfunction.

- Onset usually gradual and progressive
- Earliest feature often inability to sustain erection long enough for satisfactory intercourse
- Erectile failure may be intermittent initially
- Sudden onset often thought to indicate a psychogenic cause (but little evidence to support this)
- Preservation of spontaneous and early-morning erections does not necessarily indicate a psychogenic cause
- Loss of libido consistent with hypogonadism, but not a reliable symptom. Impotent men often understate their sex drive for a variety of reasons
- Note drug history and smoking

Investigations include serum testosterone, when there is reduced libido or suspected hypogonadism, an assessment of cardiovascular and lipid status, and a review of glycaemic control. It is now generally accepted that it is not helpful to try and determine whether erectile failure in diabetic men is of psychogenic origin.

Any features of hypogonadism

Manual dexterity—if limited, may preclude physical treatment (e.g. intracavernosal injection)

Protuberant abdomen

External genitalia
- Presence of phimosis, balanitis, Peyronie's disease
- Testicular volume

Cardiovascular disease (leg pulses, iliac and femoral bruits

FIGURE 22.7
Key physical signs to note on examination of the patient with erectile dysfunction.

Serum testosterone (ideally taken at 9 AM)—if libido reduced or hypogonadism suspected

Serum prolactin and luteinizing hormone (LH)—if serum testosterone subnormal

Assessment of cardiovascular status if clinically indicated
- Electrocardiography (ECG)
- Serum lipids

Glycosylated haemoglobin, serum electrolytes if clinically indicated

FIGURE 22.8
Investigation of erectile dysfunction in diabetes.

General measures
- Improve diabetic control
- Reduce alcohol intake
- Withdraw causative drugs
- Correct endocrine problems

Discussion and counselling (ideally with partner)
- Informal
- Formal sex or psychological therapy not usually necessary

Drugs
- Oral sildenafil or other phosphodiesterase inhibitor

FIGURE 22.9
First-line treatment of impotence in diabetic men.

General treatment measures include improving glycaemic control, reducing alcohol intake, withdrawing causative drugs when possible, and a discussion about the causes of erectile dysfunction in diabetes. Patients should stop smoking, though there is as yet no evidence that this improves erectile function in diabetes. There is generally no need for a psycho-sexual counsellor, except when there is a failing relationship or loss of attraction between partners, severe anxiety (including performance anxiety) and fear of intimacy. Most diabetic men with impotence should be offered as first-line therapy oral treatment with sildenafil (Viagra) or another phosphodiesterase type 5 (PDE-5) inhibitor. These agents act by inhibiting the breakdown of cGMP (the second messenger of NO, see Fig. 22.3) by PDE-5, and hence enhance erections under conditions of sexual stimulation.

As sildenafil interacts with organic nitrates to cause acute hypotension, concurrent use with nitrates is contraindicated absolutely. Sildenafil is generally taken 1 hour before intended sexual activity (usually 50 mg starting dose; most men routinely require 100 mg, with 25 mg in older patients or those with renal or hepatic impairment). It is effective in about 50–60% of diabetic men and is generally well tolerated. The most common side-effects are headache, dyspepsia and flushing.

Sildenafil (Viagra)

- Prevents cGMP breakdown by inhibiting PDE-5
- Natural erectile response to sexual stimulation
- Effective in ~60% of diabetic patients
- Should not be given to those treated with nitrates

More recently introduced PDE-5 inhibitors include vardenafil and tadalafil.

FIGURE 22.10
Sildenafil (Viagra).

Other options for treating erectile dysfunction in diabetes include oral apomorphine, a dopamine agonist for which a sublingual preparation has been introduced recently. Nausea is its main side-effect. Intracavernosal self-injection of prostaglandin E (alprostadil) is effective, but has a high discontinuation rate in the long term; there is a small risk of priapism (sustained unwanted erection), which must be treated within 6 hours by aspiration of blood from the corpus cavernosum. Transurethral alprostadil (MUSE) is an alternative that avoids penile injection (which some men find objectionable). Penile pain is reported in about 10% and, as with injection, the long-term usage is disappointing.

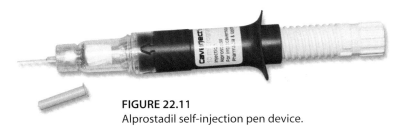

FIGURE 22.11
Alprostadil self-injection pen device.

Vacuum devices have been in use since the 1970s. A translucent tube is placed over the penis and air pumped out to draw blood into the erectile tissue. A constriction band around the base of the penis maintains the erection.

There remains a limited role for the surgical insertion of penile prostheses for men in whom conventional treatments have failed.

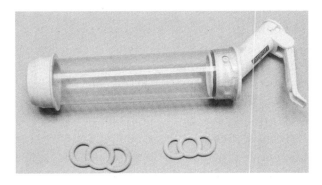

FIGURE 22.12
A typical vacuum device with constriction rings.

Sexual dysfunction seems to be much less common in diabetic women than in men, but there is an increased risk of vaginal dryness and impaired sexual arousal. The pathophysiology is poorly understood and (unlike in men) there does not seem to be a clear relationship with autonomic neuropathy. Menstrual irregularities are also common in diabetic women, particularly in those with obesity and poor glycaemic control. Insulin requirements alter around the time of menstruation in about 40% of diabetic women; the majority need more insulin, but about 10% require less. Type 2 diabetes and impaired glucose tolerance (IGT) are common in women with the polycystic ovary syndrome (PCOS) – features of which include oligomenorrhoea or amenorrhoea, polycystic ovaries (on ultrasound examination), obesity, hirsutism and raised circulating androgen levels. Both type 2 diabetes with IGT and PCOS share an association with insulin resistance. It is thought that hyperinsulinaemia stimulates androgen synthesis and thecal hypertrophy in the ovary.

Sexual problems in diabetic women

• Vaginal dryness

• Menstrual irregularities

• Infection

• Contraception

• Hormone replacement therapy

• Pregnancy

• Association with polycystic ovary syndrome (PCOS)

FIGURE 22.13
Sexual problems in diabetic women.

Genitourinary infections are common in diabetic women. Vaginal candidiasis is especially frequent in poorly controlled subjects; it can be irritating and painful and may interfere with sexual activity. Treatment involves improving control, and local or oral antifungal agents, including fluconazole. Other genital infections, such as genital herpes and pelvic inflammatory disease, occur in diabetic women, but possibly no more frequently than in the general female population. However, urinary tract infections are frequent in patients with poorly controlled diabetes, and especially in those with autonomic neuropathy and bladder distension.

Genitourinary infections in diabetic women

• Vaginal candidiasis

• Vaginal warts, herpes

• Pelvic inflammatory disease

• Urinary tract infections

FIGURE 22.14
Genitourinary infections in diabetic women.

Contraceptive advice is essential in diabetes, because unplanned pregnancies in the poorly controlled patient carry an increased risk of fetal morbidity and mortality. In many countries, the preferred method of contraception for women with diabetes is the oral contraceptive pill – which has the lowest failure rate (apart from sterilization). On the available evidence, low-dose (<30 μg oestradiol) combined oral contraceptives can be used safely in type 1 and 2 diabetes; all women who take the pill should have their blood pressure and serum lipids reviewed regularly. Combined pills that contain the 'third-generation' progestins, desogestrel and gestodene may carry a slightly increased risk of venous thromboembolism and are best avoided. Progesterone-only pills are also suitable for use in diabetes, but they may cause menstrual irregularities. As these are not thought to be associated with vascular disease, they are often used more in older women or in those with diabetic complications or risk factors.

FIGURE 22.15
Contraceptive use in 938 women with type 1 diabetes in the UK. OCP, oral contraceptive pill; POP, progesterone-only pill; IUCD, intrauterine contraceptive device.

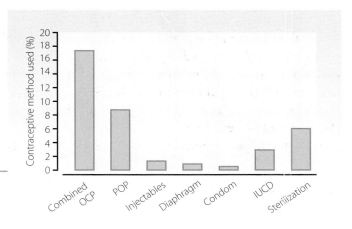

The intrauterine device (IUD) is safe and effective in diabetic women; early concerns about the risk of pelvic inflammatory disease seem to be unfounded. Condoms and diaphragms have high failure rates. However, since the advent of acquired immunodeficiency disease (AIDS), condoms have been advocated widely to reduce the transmission of sexually transmitted diseases (STDs). For high-risk individuals, many genitourinary clinics recommend a combination of oral contraceptive pill and condom to minimize the risk of both pregnancy and STD.

Method	If method is used correctly	General outcome of method
Withdrawal	20	40
Rhythm method	10	25
Spermicides	10	20
Diaphragm	5	10
Condom	5	10
IUD	4	4
Contraceptive pill	<1	2
Vasectomy	<1	<1
Tubal sterilization	<1	<1

FIGURE 22.16
The chances of pregnancy with various contraceptive methods: the number of women who become pregnant for each 100 couples who use the method for 1 year is indicated. If no method is used, 80/100 women become pregnant per year.

Hormone replacement therapy (HRT) is an established treatment for symptoms of the menopause and for those with osteoporosis. HRT does not worsen glucose tolerance and lipid profiles, and may even improve them. However, HRT has been used with some reluctance in diabetic women, possibly because of concerns about the risks of thromboembolism in the already procoagulant state of diabetes. There is insufficient evidence to recommend HRT to reduce cardiovascular risk – an important potential indication, as post-menopausal diabetic women have a considerably increased risk of ischaemic heart disease. Indeed, a recent study of post-menopausal Danish nurses reported an increased risk of all-cause death, ischaemic heart disease and myocardial infarction in diabetic women who take HRT. Long-term use of HRT in diabetes therefore needs further study.

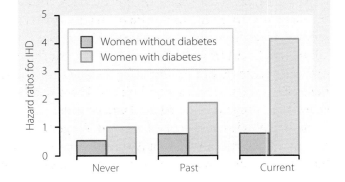

FIGURE 22.17
Hazard ratios for ischaemic heart disease (IHD) associated with the use of hormone replacement therapy stratified on diabetic status.

Disordered gastrointestinal motor function is common in both type 1 and type 2 diabetes. Potential problems include symptoms, malnutrition, poor glycaemic control, delayed absorption of orally administered drugs, and postprandial hypotension. Traditionally, this has been attributed to irreversible autonomic neuropathy, but acute changes in blood glucose also play a role. For example, hyperglycaemia delays gastric emptying, slows gall-bladder contraction and small intestinal transit, and inhibits colonic reflexes. On the other hand, hypoglycaemia accelerates gastric emptying. The mechanisms are unclear.

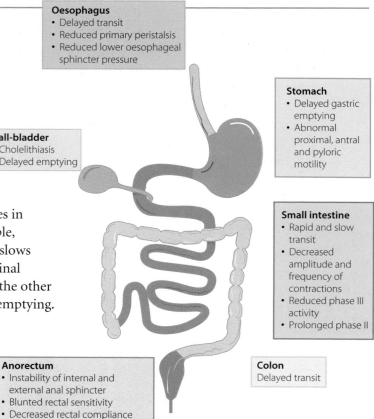

Oesophagus
• Delayed transit
• Reduced primary peristalsis
• Reduced lower oesophageal sphincter pressure

Stomach
• Delayed gastric emptying
• Abnormal proximal, antral and pyloric motility

Gall-bladder
• Cholelithiasis
• Delayed emptying

Small intestine
• Rapid and slow transit
• Decreased amplitude and frequency of contractions
• Reduced phase III activity
• Prolonged phase II

Anorectum
• Instability of internal and external anal sphincter
• Blunted rectal sensitivity
• Decreased rectal compliance
• Alterations in rectal reflex activity

Colon
Delayed transit

FIGURE 23.1
Motility disorders associated with diabetes at various levels of the gastrointestinal tract.

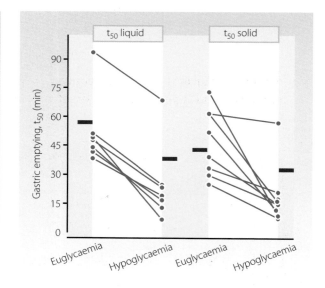

FIGURE 23.2
Dose-dependent effect of hyperglycaemia on postprandial gall-bladder contraction in healthy subjects. *$P < 0.05$ compared with 4 mmol/L; †$P < 0.05$ compared with 4, 8 and 12 mmol/L.

FIGURE 23.3
Effect of insulin-induced hypoglycaemia on gastric emptying (50% emptying, t_{50}) of 200 g solid (processed beef and vegetables) and liquid (150 mL 10% dextrose in water) in eight uncomplicated type 1 diabetic subjects. (Mean ± SD.)

Gastrointestinal symptoms, such as abdominal pain, discomfort or fullness, heartburn, difficulty in swallowing, diarrhoea and constipation, are common in diabetes, possibly more than in the general population. However, there is little relationship between the symptoms and either demonstrable motor dysfunction (e.g. gastric emptying time) or autonomic neuropathy. Among the additional factors that influence symptoms are hyperglycaemia (which increases the perception of visceral sensation, such as gut fullness), and drugs such as metformin and acarbose (which can cause diarrhoea and faecal incontinence); there is also a strong association between gastrointestinal symptoms and psychological stress.

FIGURE 23.4
Prevalence of gastrointestinal symptoms in diabetes mellitus and controls, based on a population-based study of 423 diabetic patients (22 type 1, 401 type 2).

Symptoms	Prevalence rate (%)		Adjusted odds ratios with 95% CI
	Controls (n = 8185)	Diabetic patients (n = 423)	
Abdominal pain/discomfort	10.8	13.5	1.63 (1.21–2.20)
Postprandial fullness	5.2	8.6	2.07 (1.43–3.01)
Heartburn	10.8	13.5	1.38 (1.03–1.86)
Nausea	3.5	5.2	2.31 (1.45–3.68)
Vomiting	1.1	1.7	2.51 (1.12–5.66)
Dysphagia	1.7	5.4	2.71 (1.69–4.36)
Faecal incontinence	0.8	2.6	2.74 (1.40–5.37)
Oesophageal symptoms	11.5	15.4	1.44 (1.09–1.91)
Upper dysmotility symptoms	15.3	18.2	1.75 (1.34–2.29)
Any bowel symptom	18.9	26.0	1.84 (1.46–2.33)
Diarrhoea symptoms	10.0	15.6	2.06 (1.56–2.74)
Constipation symptoms	9.2	11.4	1.54 (1.12–2.13)

Oesophageal transit is delayed in about 30–50% of diabetic subjects (mostly because of impaired peristalsis) and is associated with dysphagia, heartburn and chest pain. Endoscopy is required to exclude other disorders, such as carcinoma and candidiasis. Minimal symptoms do not require treatment; indeed, no treatment, including prokinetic drugs, has yet been shown clearly effective for more severe symptoms attributable to hypomotility.

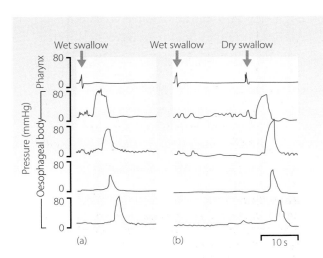

FIGURE 23.5
Wet swallow-induced oesophageal peristalsis in a healthy subject (a) and in a patient with long-standing insulin-dependent diabetes (b). In the diabetic subject, the swallow-induced peristaltic wave has insufficient force to propel the water bolus distally (failed peristalsis). A subsequent dry swallow is associated with normal peristalsis, and clears the oesophagus.

Delayed gastric emptying (gastroparesis) of a modest extent occurs in up to 50% of long-standing diabetic subjects. Symptoms of gastroparesis are characteristically worse postprandially, and include nausea, vomiting, abdominal discomfort and/or fullness and anorexia. Glycaemic control is usually poor. Examination can show epigastric distension and a succussion splash if the stomach is grossly dilated. A plain abdominal radiograph classically shows a 'ground glass' appearance in the upper abdomen. Scintigraphy is the standard method for measuring gastric emptying; ideally, this should be performed at euglycaemia and with dual isotope assessment of both solid and liquid emptying (Fig. 23.3). Endoscopy is often required to exclude other causes of gastroparesis and pathology, such as gastric outlet disorder or small intestinal obstruction and mucosal disorders. Some drugs can delay gastric emptying (morphine, anticholinergics, nicotine and dopaminergics).

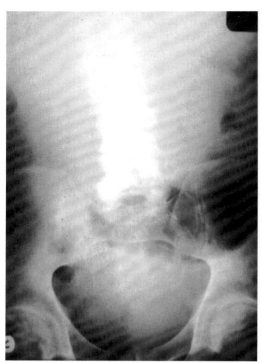

FIGURE 23.6
Plain abdominal radiograph showing uniform 'ground glass' appearance in the upper abdomen caused by the greatly distended fluid-filled stomach of gastroparesis.

General measures
Maintain good glycaemic control.
• Eat small, frequent meals; avoid high-fibre foods
Oral prokinetic drugs
• Cisapride (restricted use)
• Metoclopramide
• Domperidone
• Erythromycin
Endoscopy indicated if:
Haematemesis (usually due to Mallory–Weiss tear)
Other pathology or bezoar suspected
Severe episodes
Hospital admission
Intravenous rehydration
Intravenous prokinetic drugs
• Metoclopramide 10 mg 4-hourly
• Erythromycin 200 mg (3 mg/kg) 4-hourly
Nasogastric tube and drainage
Nutrition
• Intravenous
• Intrajejunal, via gastrostomy (PEG tube)
Surgical drainage procedures as a last resort

Treatment of symptomatic gastroparesis can be difficult; it involves improving glycaemic control, eating small meals often, and administration of prokinetic drugs such as domperidone, metoclopramide and erythromycin (possibly better given as a suspension). Cisapride was until recently the prokinetic drug of choice, but it can cause cardiotoxicity and its use is restricted in many countries. Severely affected patients may need admission to hospital for intravenous fluid repletion, control of diabetes and possibly drainage of the stomach *via* a nasogastric tube. Placement of a feeding jejunostomy to maintain nutrition may be required, but surgery is to be avoided if possible. There has been renewed interest in gastric electrical stimulation ('pacing') for intractable gastroparesis, but more trials are needed.

FIGURE 23.7
Management of diabetic gastroparesis.

Autonomic neuropathy and sometimes colonization of the hypomotile small bowel by colonic bacteria contribute to 'diabetic diarrhoea', but other factors probably play a role. Classically, the diarrhoea is intermittent and often worse at night. Bouts that last several days may be followed by remissions. The diagnosis is by exclusion, and other possible causes of diarrhoea, such as drugs (metformin, acarbose, antibiotics and alcohol), chronic pancreatic disease and coeliac disease, must be eliminated.

Diarrhoea

- Usually long-standing, poorly controlled diabetes
- Other evidence of autonomic neuropathy
- Diarrhoea often intermittent
- Diarrhoea often nocturnal

FIGURE 23.8
Diarrhoea in diabetic patients.

Treatment of diabetic diarrhoea is by opioids (e.g. loperamide), or a broad-spectrum antibiotic if bacterial overgrowth is suspected or proved. Troublesome diarrhoea, especially when watery, may respond to the α-adrenergic agonists, clonidine or limidine. The long-acting somatostatin analogue, octreotide, may be helpful when other measures have failed.

Agent	Dosage
Opioid derivatives	
• Codeine phosphate	30 mg, three to four times daily
• Loperamide hydrochloride	2 mg, three to four times daily
Broad-spectrum antibiotics (for bacterial overgrowth)	
• Oxytetracycline	250 mg, four times daily — for 5–7 days
• Erythromycin	250 mg, four times daily
α₂-adrenergic agent	
• Clonidine	0.3–0.6 mg, twice daily
Somatostatin analogue	
• Octreotide	50–100 μg subcutaneously, two to three times daily

FIGURE 23.9
Drug treatments for diabetic diarrhoea.

Constipation is also common in diabetic patients with autonomic neuropathy and poor glycaemic control, though it is usually mild. A thorough history should be taken, including that of drug intake (many narcotics, antihypertensives and antidepressants can cause constipation). Thyroid function and serum calcium and potassium levels should be assessed to exclude metabolic disorder. Other serious pathology, such as colonic carcinoma, must be excluded by rectal examination, proctosigmoidoscopy, colonoscopy or barium enema. If constipation requires treatment, fibre and bulking agents are the first choice; stimulant laxatives (e.g. senna), osmotic laxatives (e.g. lactulose) or prokinetic drugs are also usually effective.

Constipation

- Common (up to ~80% of those with neuropathy)
- Usually mild
- Tends to be neglected
- Exclude metabolic causes, drugs and pathology

FIGURE 23.10
Constipation in diabetic patients.

SKIN AND CONNECTIVE TISSUE DISORDERS IN DIABETES

24

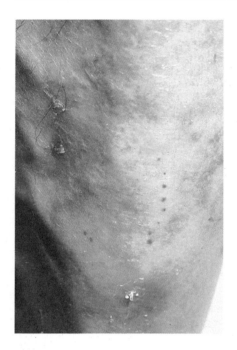

The skin condition associated most commonly with diabetes is diabetic dermopathy or 'shin spots', which usually occur in clusters in up to 50% of patients, especially those over the age of 50 years (one or two such lesions also occur in up to 3% of non-diabetic people). Early lesions are oval, red papules, up to 1 cm in diameter. They slowly become well-circumscribed, atrophic, brown and scaly scars. The usual site is the pretibial region (hence shin spots), but forearms, thighs and bony prominences may be involved. There is no effective treatment, but the spots tend to resolve over 1–2 years.

FIGURE 24.1
Diabetic dermopathy, or 'shin spots'.

Necrobiosis lipoidica diabeticorum (NLD) is more common in diabetes than in the general population, but is still rare, occurring in about 0.3% of diabetic subjects. It usually develops in young adulthood or early middle life, with three times more women affected than men. The shin is the usual site, where typical chronic lesions are irregularly shaped, indurated plaques with central atrophy. The surface is shiny with telangiectatic vessels that cross a yellowish waxy central area. Ulceration occurs in about 25%. NDL lesions are partially or completely anaesthetic.

FIGURE 24.2
Necrobiosis lipoidica diabeticorum (NLD). (a) An early lesion on an ankle, showing the erythematous stage. (b) A long-standing patch of NLD. Note the typical yellow, atrophic appearance with telangiectasia.

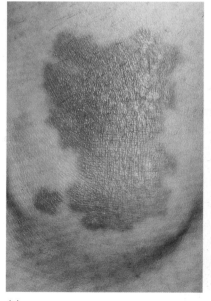

(a)

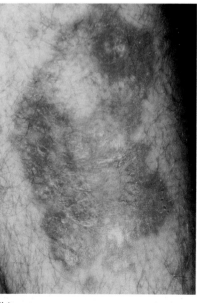

(b)

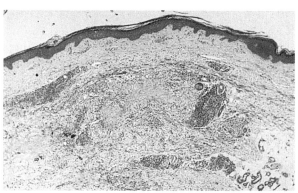

The aetiology of NLD is unknown. Histologically, there is hyaline degeneration of collagen in the dermis ('necrobiosis'), surrounded by fibrosis, and with a diffuse histiocytic infiltrate and frequently a granulomatous reaction of giant cells similar to those seen with sarcoidosis. Treatment is unsatisfactory, with no response to improved glycaemic control. Corticosteroids may improve early NLD, but should not be used in chronic atrophic lesions. Cosmetic camouflage seems the best option in most cases.

FIGURE 24.3
Histological features of necrobiosis lipoidica diabeticorum (NLD), showing degeneration of the collagen ('necrobiosis'), associated with fibrosis and a histiocytic infiltrate. Haematoxylin and eosin stain, original magnification ×40.

Cheiroarthropathy

The skin is generally thickened in diabetes, probably because of glycation of dermal collagen and cross-linking to form advanced glycation end products (AGEs). Usually, this is clinically insignificant, but the combination of thickened, tight and waxy skin with limited joint mobility (cheiroarthropathy) is present in 30–40% of type 1 diabetic patients. This can lead to stiff and painful fingers. Thickening over the dorsum of the fingers is termed 'Garrod's knuckle pads'.

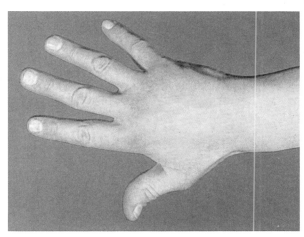

FIGURE 24.4
Garrod's knuckle pads.

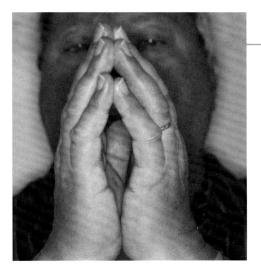

A typical sign of the 'diabetic hand syndrome' is the 'prayer sign', in which limited joint mobility because of thickened and waxy skin does not allow the patient to press both palms together.

FIGURE 24.5
The 'prayer sign'.

219

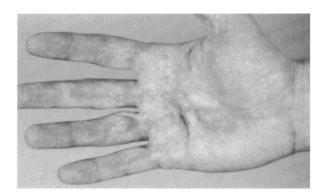

Dupuytren's contracture occurs in up to half of diabetic patients, especially in the elderly and those with long-standing disease; it often co-exists with cheiroarthropathy.

FIGURE 24.6
Dupuytren's contracture.

'Trigger finger' occurs when there is intermittent locking of the finger, associated with stenosing flexor tenosynovitis, which is often seen in diabetes. A nodular swelling and thickening of the tendon sheath can often be palpated. It responds to steroid injection. Adhesive capsulitis of the shoulder (sometimes called 'frozen shoulder') is a further non-articular fibrosing disorder that occurs more commonly in diabetes than in the general population, and is characterized by pain and limitation of movement. Analgesics and physiotherapy should be tried first, and intra-articular steroids may be given later.

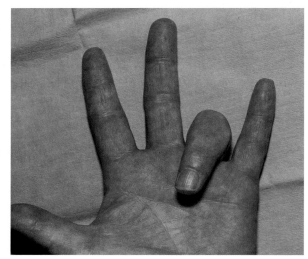

FIGURE 24.7
Trigger finger in a diabetic patient.

Acanthosis nigricans is a hyperpigmented velvety overgrowth of the epidermis, usually in the flexural areas of the axilla, groin and neck. It is associated with various causes of insulin resistance and hyperinsulinaemia (such as genetic and autoimmune insulin receptor defects, and lipoatrophic diabetes, see Chapter 8), possibly because raised circulating insulin levels act *via* insulin-like growth factor-1 (IGF-1) receptors in the skin to stimulate growth.

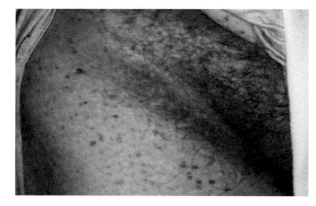

FIGURE 24.8
Acanthosis nigricans.

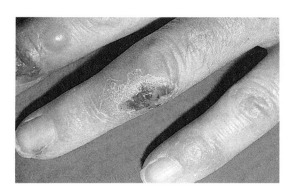

Diabetic bullae are rare and appear as tense blisters on a non-inflammatory base, most often on the feet or lower legs, followed by the hands. They tend to heal over a few weeks.

FIGURE 24.9
Diabetic bullae.

Various other skin problems are associated with long-standing diabetes, but are not specific to diabetes. These include bacterial infections (e.g. boils and sepsis caused by *Staphylococcus aureus*), *Candida albicans* infections (e.g. vulvovaginitis, balanitis, intertrigo and chronic paronychia) and tinea (dermatophyte fungal infections). Note also the occurrence of neuropathic and ischaemic foot ulcers in diabetes (see Chapter 21), and the dry skin caused by decreased sweating with autonomic neuropathy.

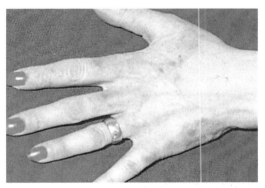

FIGURE 24.10
Tinea manus, showing the characteristic erythematous, scaly margin.

Chronic paronychia presents with swelling and erythema around the nail-folds, often with a discharge. Severe involvement may produce oncholysis. Treatment is by keeping the fingers dry and the use of antifungal drugs; systemic drugs such as fluconazole, rather than topical administration, may be necessary.

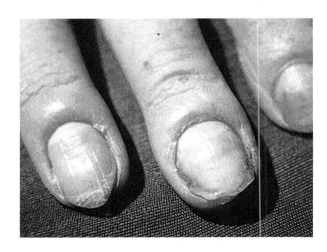

FIGURE 24.11
Chronic paronychia caused by *Candida albicans*.

Cutaneous side-effects of antidiabetic drugs include insulin-induced lipoatrophy and lipohypertrophy (see Chapter 10), and the now rare localized and systemic allergic insulin reactions such as urticaria and pruritus. Skin reactions from sulphonylurea drugs are more frequent with first-generation agents such as chlorpropamide, and include maculopapular rashes and erythema multiforme. The severe form of the latter is Stevens–Johnson syndrome with target lesions and blistering ulceration of the mucous membranes of the mouth and the eyes (always seek ophthalmic advice). Chlorpropamide causes facial flushing after drinking alcohol.

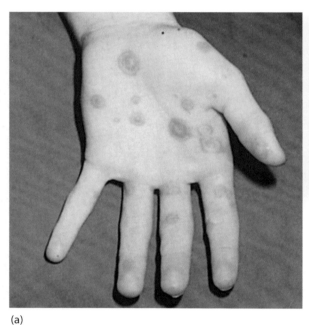

(a)

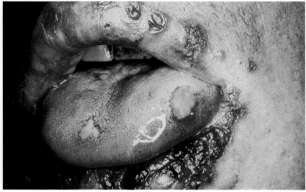

(b)

FIGURE 24.12
Erythema multiforme, showing (a) typical target lesions and (b) mouth ulceration in Stevens–Johnson syndrome, the severe form of erythema multiforme. The eyes are also often involved.

Particular groups of diabetic patients are at risk of different psychological problems. Many children show remarkable resilience to the diagnosis of diabetes, but about one-third have some temporary psychological distress, mostly 'adjustment disorders' such as difficulty in sleeping, depression, social withdrawal and anxiety. This generally subsides within 6 months. Surprisingly little is known about psychological problems in adults with recent-onset diabetes.

Diabetic group	Psychological problem
Children and adolescents at onset of diabetes (little known about adults with recent-onset diabetes)	Temporary adjustment disorder— somatic complaints, social withdrawal, sleeping disorder, anxiety, depression
Older adults with established diabetes, especially when hospitalized, in females and those with past psychopathology	Higher frequency of depression (but comparable to other chronic illnesses)
Patients with macrovascular disease, chronic foot ulceration and proliferative retinopathy	Depression, poor quality of life, psychological distress
Children with repeated hypoglycaemia (especially when onset of diabetes is < 5 years of age)	Mild impairment of cognitive functioning —visuospatial/verbal defects, etc.
Later-onset children and adolescents	Verbal IQ and academic achievement lowered
Adults with chronic hyperglycaemia	Defects in psychomotor tasks, attention, learning and memory

FIGURE 25.1
Diabetic groups at risk of developing psychological problems.

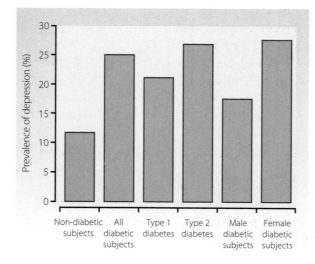

FIGURE 25.2
The increased prevalence of depression in diabetic compared with non-diabetic subjects. The data are from a meta-analysis of 42 studies.

Most children and adolescents function well psychologically during the course of their diabetes, although there is an increased frequency of psychiatric disorders by 10 years' diabetes duration, mainly severe depression and anxiety. In adults with diabetes, depression and anxiety are about twice as high as in the general population. The highest rates are in hospitalized patients, those with macrovascular disease, chronic foot ulceration, proliferative retinopathy and previous psychopathology; females are more susceptible than males. There is only a weak relationship between metabolic control and mood disorder. Depression may precede and predict the development of type 2 diabetes.

The features of moderate or severe depression should be recognized by diabetologists, although cases are often missed in the setting of a busy diabetic clinic and because some symptoms of depression overlap with those of diabetes itself (e.g. weight loss, lethargy and loss of libido).

Depressed mood most of the day, nearly every day (also anxiety, irritability)
Loss of interest or enjoyment
Decreased appetite and weight loss
Loss of libido
Insomnia (early morning wakening, initial insomnia or interrupted sleep) or hypersomnia
Fatigue or loss of energy
Psychomotor retardation
Poor concentration
Reduced self-esteem and confidence
Thoughts of hopelessness, worthlessness or guilt
Suicidal ideas or attempts

FIGURE 25.3
Depressive symptoms. Symptoms must be present for at least 2 weeks to make the diagnosis.

Anxiety is also more frequent in those with diabetes. Some of the symptoms of anxiety, such as sweating, tremor, palpitations, nausea and headache, may be confused with hypoglycaemia by both patients and doctors. Fear of hypoglycaemia is a major problem and may be severe enough to meet the criteria for phobia. Fear of needles can also cause significant anxiety in diabetes. Anxiety may exacerbate hyperglycaemia or cause hypoglycaemia in diabetes through the effects of stress hormones, such as catecholamines and cortisol, and by the disruption of self-care behaviours.

Emotion	Fear, anxiety, panic
Physical symptoms	Sweating, tremor, tachycardia, breathlessness, muscular tension, difficulty swallowing, numbness, tingling, nausea, dizziness, dry mouth, headache, epigastric discomfort, etc.
Thoughts	Catastrophic thoughts, e.g. 'I'm going to die', 'I'm going to collapse', 'I'm going to make a fool of myself', 'I'm going to lose control'
	Overestimation of danger
Behaviour	Avoidance of specific situations
	Escape from situations
	Safety-seeking behaviour, e.g. never going into situation alone

FIGURE 25.4
Typical anxiety symptoms.

Children diagnosed under the age of 5 or 6 years are most at risk of cognitive dysfunction; initial defects are in visuospatial ability (copying, solving jigsaws), which by adolescence progresses to impaired learning and memory, verbal ability, and school achievement. The cause may be hypoglycaemia, which is more common in young children than in those >5 years of age because the developing brain is especially sensitive to hypoglycaemic damage. Repeated hypoglycaemia in adults does not seem to impair cognition.

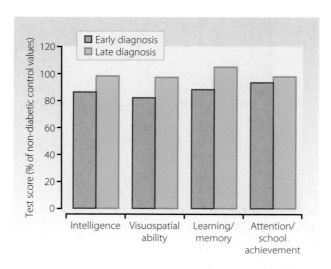

FIGURE 25.5
The impairment of cognitive ability in 125 adolescents with type 1 diabetes diagnosed at <5 years of age (early diagnosis), compared with those diagnosed at >5 years of age (late diagnosis).

In adults with type 1 diabetes and older adults with type 2 diabetes, chronic hyperglycaemia is associated with defects in psychomotor tasks, attention, learning and memory. This may be associated with distal symmetrical neuropathy, and it has been postulated that the metabolic mechanisms that lead to diabetic peripheral neuropathy (see Chapters 14 and 17) may also cause a 'central neuropathy'.

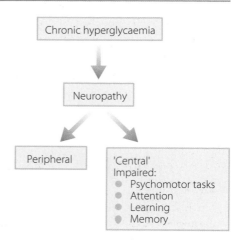

FIGURE 25.6
Hyperglycaemia may cause a central neuropathy with psychological impairment.

Treatment of depression begins with general measures such as sympathetic discussion, advice about improving glycaemic control and attention to specific causes of anxiety, such as fear of blindness, infertility, impotence, amputation, etc. Sleep disorders are common and may be helped by taking regular exercise and avoiding daytime naps, large meals, tobacco, alcohol and caffeine-containing drinks in the evening. Moderate or severe depression may require antidepressant drugs.

Treatment of depression

- General measures (diabetic control, sympathetic discussion, specific anxieties, attention to sleep disorders)

- Anti-depressant drugs for non-responders and for moderate/severe depression

- Consider cognitive behaviour therapy

FIGURE 25.7
Treatment of depression.

Antidepressant drugs are comparably effective in diabetes but selective serotonin reuptake inhibitors (e.g. fluoxetine, sertraline) have the advantages of low cardiotoxicity, greater safety in overdose, less sedation, lack of weight gain and lack of anticholinergic side-effects. Tricyclic antidepressants can raise blood glucose levels, induce sedation and weight gain, and have some cardiotoxicity and anticholinergic side-effects (e.g. dry mouth, blurred vision, hesitancy or urinary retention). Some tricyclics, such imipramine, nortryptiline and lofepramine, have weaker sedative properties and are useful in withdrawn or apathetic patients; tricyclic drugs with sedative action (e.g. amitriptyline) are more suitable for agitated or anxious patients. Monoamine oxidase inhibitors are currently little used. Cognitive behaviour therapy is also effective, but therapists should be familiar with diabetes and its problems so that diabetes-specific issues are addressed.

First choice:

Selective serotonin reuptake inhibitors (e.g. fluoxetine, sertraline)

Second choice:

Tricyclic antidepressants
- Amitriptyline: sedative, use in agitated or anxious patients
- Imipramine, lofepramine: less sedative, use in withdrawn or apathetic patients

FIGURE 25.8
Antidepressant drugs.

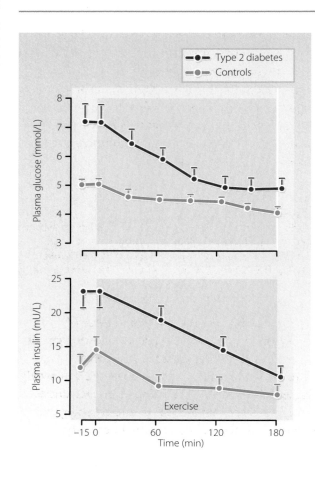

Exercise

Regular physical exercise is an important component of the management and prevention of type 2 diabetes (see Chapter 11). In type 2 diabetes, exercise does not usually cause hypoglycaemia and extra carbohydrate is unnecessary. Exercise accelerates weight loss, increases insulin sensitivity, decreases insulinaemia and improves blood glucose and lipid profiles, but it should be combined with an appropriate diet and tailored to the individual's capabilities. Everyday moderate exercise (e.g. 30–60 minutes of walking) is often sustained best. Type 2 diabetic subjects with moderate or high cardiorespiratory fitness have a long-term mortality 50–60% lower than diabetic individuals with low fitness.

FIGURE 26.1
Changes in plasma glucose and insulin concentrations during prolonged low-intensity exercise in non-obese type 2 diabetic patients. The exercise (30–35% of maximal) was performed after an overnight fast. The fall in endogenous insulin secretion diminishes the risk of hypoglycaemia during exercise in type 2 diabetes.

In type 1 diabetes, blood glucose decreases if:

• Hyperinsulinaemia exists during exercise

• Exercise is prolonged (>30–60 min) or intensive

• Less than 3 h have elapsed since the preceding meal

• No extra snacks are taken before or during the exercise

Blood glucose generally remains unchanged if:

• Exercise is brief

• Plasma insulin concentration is normal

• Appropriate snacks are taken before and during exercise

Blood glucose increases if:

• Hypoinsulinaemia exists during exercise

• Exercise is strenuous

• Excessive carbohydrate is taken before or during exercise

In type 1 diabetes, short-term glycaemic changes during exercise depend largely on the blood insulin levels, and therefore the type of insulin used and the interval between insulin injection and exercise. For example, hyperinsulinaemia that occurs when exercise is taken shortly after the injection of short-acting insulin (and particularly when the site of insulin injection is an exercising limb) causes blood glucose to decrease. Hypoinsulinaemia that coincides with exercise taken many hours after insulin injection may cause blood glucose to rise after exercise. Other factors that determine the effects of exercise are the intensity of the exercise and the intake of food.

FIGURE 26.2
Factors that determine the glycaemic response to acute exercise in type 1 diabetes.

HANDBOOK OF DIABETES 3RD EDITION

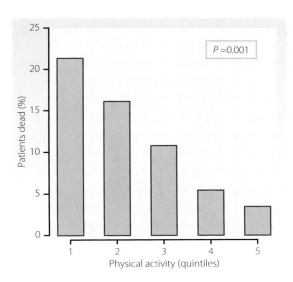

Interestingly, most studies have not found that exercise improves overall long-term glycaemic control in type 1 diabetes, perhaps because patients tend to consume extra carbohydrate to prevent hypoglycaemia. However, as with type 2 diabetes, type 1 patients who exercise regularly have lower long-term morbidity and mortality compared with their sedentary counterparts.

FIGURE 26.3
Proportion of men who died during a 7-year follow-up period among 548 type 1 diabetic patients, stratified according to their physical activity quintile. Quintile cut-offs were <398, 398–1000, 1000–2230, 2230–4228 and >4228 kcal/week.

Monitor glycaemia before, during and after exercise as necessary

Avoid hypoglycaemia during exercise by:
• Taking 20–40 g extra carbohydrate before and hourly during exercise
• Avoiding heavy exercise during peak insulin injection
• Using non-exercising sites for insulin injection
• Reducing preinjection insulin dosages by 30–50% if necessary

After prolonged exercise, monitor glycaemia and take extra carbohydrate to avoid delayed hypoglycaemia

FIGURE 26.4
Guidelines for exercise in type 1 diabetes.

Type 1 diabetic patients can reduce the risk of hypoglycaemia during exercise by following specific guidelines, which include close blood glucose monitoring, extra carbohydrate taken before and hourly during exercise, avoiding exercising muscle territories used for injection (such as the legs) and reducing the pre-exercise insulin dose by 30–50% if necessary.

Drugs

Numerous drugs can affect diabetic control, and cause hyper- or hypoglycaemia by interfering with insulin secretion or action or both, or by interacting with antidiabetic agents.

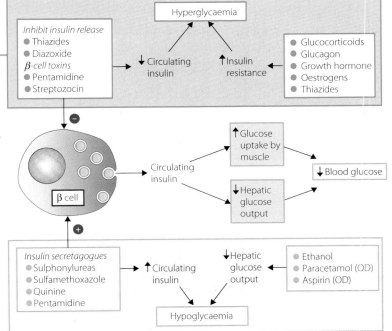

FIGURE 26.5
General mechanisms of drug-induced hyper- and hypoglycaemia. OD, overdose.

HANDBOOK OF DIABETES 3RD EDITION

Hyperglycaemia can be caused or worsened by many drugs. Corticosteroids, which are widely prescribed for numerous medical conditions, have an especially potent diabetogenic effect and act by inducing insulin resistance. Dosages equivalent to ≥30 mg/day of prednisolone are especially likely to raise blood glucose in diabetic patients, and may cause glucose intolerance or overt diabetes in previously normoglycaemic individuals. Oral contraceptives rarely worsen diabetic control; the risks of hyperglycaemia are highest with the (now obsolete) high-dose oestrogen pills, combined pills that contain the progestogen levonorgestrel and in women with a history of gestational diabetes. High-dose thiazide diuretics (e.g. ≥5 mg/day of bendrofluazide) cause insulin resistance and impair insulin secretion, whereas lower dosages (2.5 mg/day bendrofluazide) – which are still effective in controlling blood pressure – do not. Diabetogenic drugs that damage the β cell include pentamidine (an antiprotozoal agent) and ciclosporin.

Potentially potent effects	Minor or no effects
Glucocorticoids	Oral contraceptives
Oral contraceptives	• Progestogen-only pills
• High-dose oestrogen	Thiazides (low dosages)*
• Levonorgestrel in combination pills	Loop diuretics
Thiazide diuretics (high dosages)*	ACE inhibitors
β_2-adrenoceptor antagonists	Calcium-channel blockers
β_2-adrenoceptor agonists	α_1-adrenoceptor antagonists
• Salbutamol	Growth hormone (physiological
• Ritodrine	doses)
Atypical antipsychotics	Somatostatin analogues†
• Clozapine	Selective serotonin re-uptake
• Olanzapine	inhibitors
HIV protease inhibitors	
• Indinavir, nelfinavir and others	
Others	
• Pentamidine	
• Streptozocin	
• Diazoxide	
• Ciclosporin	
• Tacrolimus	

ACE, angiotensin-converting enzyme; HIV, human immunodeficiency virus.

*'High' and 'low' dosages of thiazides correspond to ≥5 mg/day and ≤2.5 mg/day of bendroflumethiazide, respectively.

†Somatostatin analogues may induce hyperglycaemia in type 2 but not type 1 diabetes.

FIGURE 26.6
Drugs that cause or exacerbate hyperglycaemia.

Management of corticosteroid-induced diabetes depends largely on the degree of hyperglycaemia. Diet or diet and a sulphonylurea are often sufficient, but if significant hyperglycaemia develops, twice-daily insulin therapy should be started at a total dose of 0.5 units/kg body weight. Type 2 diabetic patients on high-dose steroids usually require the addition of a sulphonylurea (if diet treated) or insulin (if tablet treated). For those who already take insulin, the dosage may need to be increased by 50%, and then adjusted according to blood glucose values.

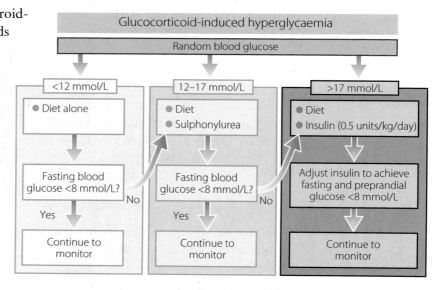

FIGURE 26.7
Treatment algorithm for glucocorticoid-induced hyperglycaemia.

Antidiabetic drugs:

- Insulins
- Sulphonylureas and glimepiride
- Repaglinide

Drugs that interact to enhance the actions of sulphonylureas

Other drugs:

- Quinine
- Quinidine
- Mefloquine
- Sulfamethoxazole (in co-trimoxazole)
- Pentamidine
- Disopyramide
- Cibenzoline
- Non-selective b-adrenoceptor antagonists
- Paracetamol (in overdosage)
- Aspirin (in overdosage)
- Ethanol

Several drugs can cause or exacerbate hypoglycaemia. Important examples are alcohol, sulfamethoxazole (combined with trimethoprim in co-trimoxazole), quinine, aspirin and paracetamol (acetaminophen) in overdosage, and the numerous drugs that enhance the action of sulphonylureas (e.g. probenecid, sulphonamides, monoamine oxidase inhibitors, chloramphenicol, fluconazole).

FIGURE 26.8
Drugs that cause or exacerbate hypoglycaemia.

Common infections with increased incidence in diabetic patients

- Urinary tract infections
- Respiratory tract infections
- Soft-tissue infections

Infections predominantly occurring in diabetic patients

- Malignant otitis externa
- Rhinocerebral mucormycosis
- Necrotizing fasciitis
- Fournier's gangrene
- Emphysematous infections
- Emphysematous cholecystitis
- Emphysematous pyelonephritis, pyelitis and cystitis
- Infections in the diabetic foot

FIGURE 26.9
Classification of infections in diabetes mellitus.

Infections

Diabetes is associated with a wide range of infections, which are more frequent than in the general population (e.g. urinary tract infections, UTI), or occur almost exclusively in diabetic subjects (e.g. malignant otitis externa), or run a different or more aggressive course in the diabetic host (e.g. some respiratory tract infections). The multiple defects in immunity in diabetes, including impaired polymorphonuclear leukocyte function, may explain the susceptibility to infection. Other contributory causes in some patients include frequent hospitalization, delayed wound healing and chronic renal failure. Common infections are UTI, respiratory tract infections and soft-tissue infections.

About 25% of diabetic women have asymptomatic bacteruria (about four times more frequent than in the non-diabetic population). *Escherichia coli* is the most common pathogen. UTI may be asymptomatic or present with dysuria, frequency or urgency (lower UTI), or flank pain, fever and vomiting (upper UTI). Perinephric abscess and papillary necrosis are rare complications.

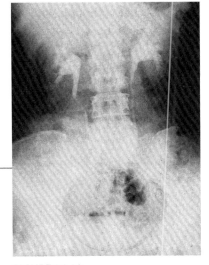

FIGURE 26.10
Acute papillary necrosis, showing loss of a papilla and a calyceal ring shadow in the left kidney.

233

With respiratory tract infections in diabetes, bacteraemia, delayed resolution and recurrence are more common than in the general population, though the overall frequency is probably no greater. Respiratory infection caused by certain micro-organisms, including *Staphylococcus aureus*, Gram-negative bacteria, *Mycobacterium tuberculosis* and *Mucor*, is more common in diabetes. Respiratory infection with *Streptococcus*, *Legionella* and influenza virus is associated with greater morbidity and mortality in diabetes. Cough and fever are the usual presenting complaints, although ketoacidosis can be the first manifestation. Deep soft-tissue infections with bacteria (e.g. pyomyositis, a muscle abscess that occurs after trauma and haematoma and is caused by *S. aureus*) and fungi (e.g. cutaneous mucormycosis) are more common in diabetes.

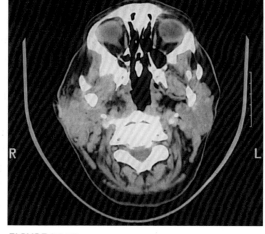

FIGURE 26.11
Necrotizing ('malignant') otitis externa. This magnetic resonance scan shows extensive soft-tissue necrosis and swelling, with early involvement of the underlying bone. The patient was a 28-year-old woman with long-standing diabetes.

Some rare infections occur predominantly in diabetic patients. Malignant otitis externa is a life-threatening condition, usually caused by *Pseudomonas aeruginosa* and most common in elderly diabetic patients. Patients present with ear discharge, severe pain and hearing impairment, with oedema, cellulitis and polypoid granulation of the auditory canal. Cranial osteomyelitis and intracranial spread of infection may occur.

Rhinocerebral mucormycosis is a rare infection caused by fungi of the *Rhizopus* or *Mucor* species, which grow best in acid media; ketoacidosis is a predisposing factor. About 50% of cases are in diabetic patients. The fungi have a predilection to invade blood vessels. Onset may be with nasal stuffiness, epistaxis and facial and ocular pain. A characteristic black necrotic eschar (scab) occurs on the nasal turbinates or palate. Complications include cavernous sinus thrombosis, cranial nerve palsies, visual loss, frontal lobe abscesses and carotid artery or jugular vein thrombosis (which cause hemiparesis).

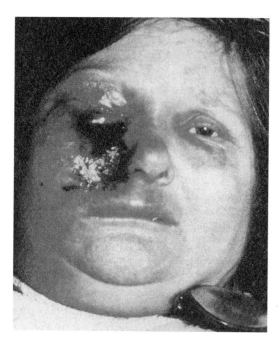

FIGURE 26.12
Rhinocerebral mucormycosis. Typical appearance, in a 45-year-old woman with poorly controlled type 1 diabetes. Periorbital and facial swelling had been present for 3–4 days before admission. Major reconstructive surgery was required.

Surgery

Surgical stress stimulates secretion of counter-regulatory hormones, such as cortisol and catecholamines, which decrease insulin sensitivity and inhibit insulin release. In insulin-deficient diabetic patients, this may cause dangerous hyperglycaemia and ketosis. In general, metabolic disturbance caused by surgery is more pronounced in type 1 diabetes. Hypoglycaemia, because of excessive anti-diabetic medication, is also a major risk of surgery in diabetic patients.

Safety and simplicity are the guiding principles of diabetes management during surgery. After preoperative assessment to confirm fitness for anaesthesia, optimization of control and liaison with the surgical and anaesthetic teams, management plans depend on whether or not the patient is insulin-treated, and on the nature and duration of surgery. In type 2 diabetic patients, long-acting sulphonylureas should be changed to short-acting agents some days before surgery, to reduce the risk of hypoglycaemia. Well-controlled, non-insulin-treated type 2 diabetic patients who undergo minor surgery can omit drugs on the morning of the operation and rely on close blood glucose monitoring during the perioperative period. In all type 1 diabetic patients and in insulin-treated or poorly controlled type 2 patients who undergo major surgery, continuous infusion of insulin and glucose is necessary to maintain metabolic control.

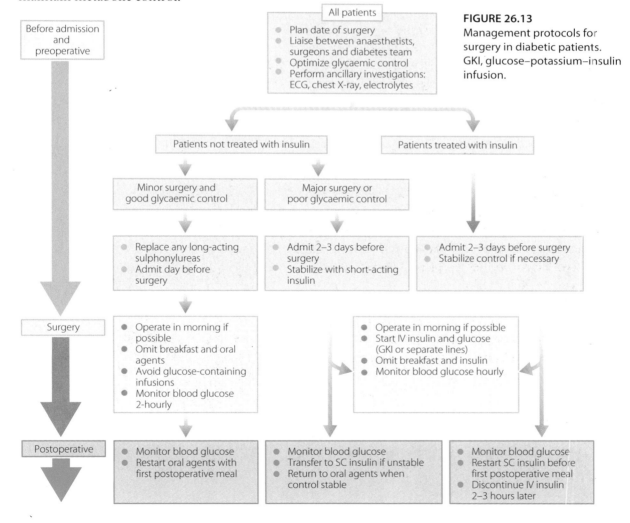

FIGURE 26.13
Management protocols for surgery in diabetic patients. GKI, glucose–potassium–insulin infusion.

235

Insulin and glucose can be given either separately or as a mixture with added potassium chloride to prevent hypokalaemia (insulin stimulates the uptake of K^+ into cells). With the simple glucose–potassium–insulin (GKI) regimen, 15 units of regular (short-acting) insulin and 10 mmol potassium chloride are added to a 500 mL bag of 10% dextrose and this mixture is infused over 5 hours. Blood glucose should be monitored 1–2 hourly, aiming for a target blood glucose range of 6–11 mmol/L. If hypo- or hyperglycaemia develop, a new infusion bag should be substituted that contains an appropriate insulin dosage (20 units if blood glucose >11 mmol/L and 10 units if <6 mmol/L).

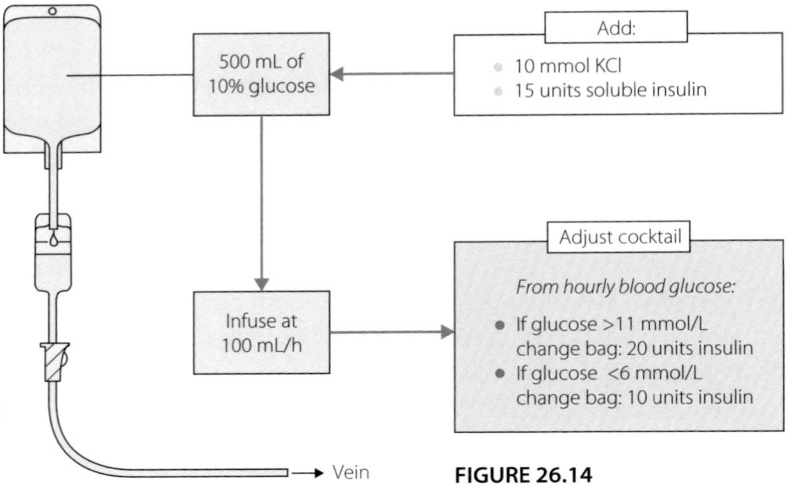

500 mL of 10% glucose

Add:
- 10 mmol KCl
- 15 units soluble insulin

Infuse at 100 mL/h

Adjust cocktail

From hourly blood glucose:
- If glucose >11 mmol/L change bag: 20 units insulin
- If glucose <6 mmol/L change bag: 10 units insulin

Vein

FIGURE 26.14
The 'GKI' (glucose–potassium–insulin) infusion. If blood glucose departs from the target range, the whole bag must be changed to deliver a more appropriate insulin dosage.

Diabetes in pregnancy poses numerous problems for both mother and fetus. In women with pre-existing diabetes, glycaemic control worsens and insulin requirements increase during pregnancy. In non-diabetic women, pregnancy may induce gestational diabetes or impaired glucose tolerance (IGT), while subjects with pre-existing glucose intolerance may become overtly diabetic. This is because pregnancy induces insulin resistance, maximal in the second and third trimesters, through the diabetogenic effects of placental hormones and progesterone. Hyperglycaemia and enhanced lipolysis (induced by insulin resistance) are probably favourable in the non-diabetic woman, as they encourage nutrient transfer to the growing fetus.

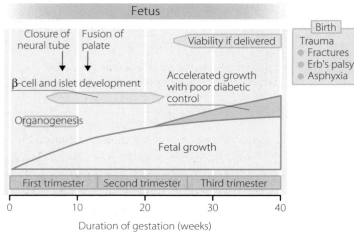

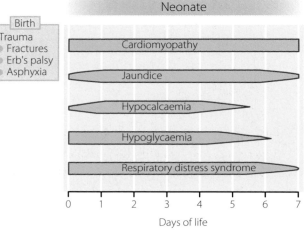

Maternal diabetes can affect the fetus adversely by causing developmental malformations, altered islet-cell development (increased insulin secretion) and accelerated and inappropriate growth (macrosomia). The respiratory distress syndrome is also about six times more frequent than in non-diabetic pregnancies and a major cause of fetal morbidity and mortality. Though the overall perinatal mortality rate has fallen in recent years, both this and the stillbirth rate remain about four times that of the non-diabetic population. Pre-eclampsia is more common in diabetic pregnancies and maternal mortality is significantly higher than in non-diabetic pregnancies.

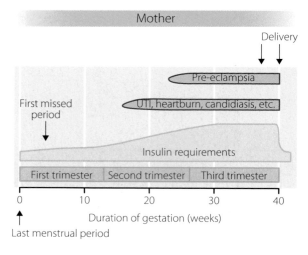

FIGURE 27.1
Impact of maternal diabetes on the fetus and neonate and the mother. UTI, urinary tract infection.

Diabetes is teratogenic, particularly in the first 8 weeks' gestation, when the major organs are forming. Defects include anencephaly, spina bifida, great-vessel abnormalities and sacral agenesis (caudal regression). The malformation rate is related to the degree of hyperglycaemia (about 30% in poorly controlled patients – 12 times the background rate), but tight control can reduce the rate. This emphasizes the vital importance of excellent control of diabetes from the time of conception – which, in practical terms, implies optimization of glycaemic control in preparation for pregnancy (see below).

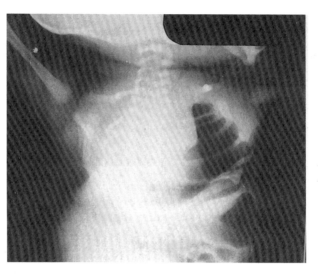

FIGURE 27.2
Radiograph of the fetus of a diabetic mother, showing sacral agenesis (the caudal regression syndrome).

Accelerated fetal growth, which leads to a macrosomic, large-for-gestational age infant, is caused by enhanced delivery of glucose and other nutrients to the fetus. This stimulates the islets and induces fetal hyperinsulinaemia, which promotes abdominal fat deposition, skeletal growth and organomegaly. Complications for these babies include birth trauma and neonatal hypoglycaemia and hypocalcaemia. Poor glycaemic control also leads to impaired production of lung surfactant and the risk of respiratory distress syndrome in the neonate.

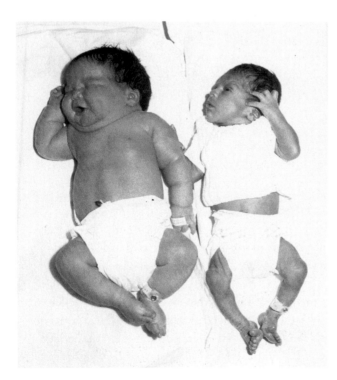

FIGURE 27.3
Left: A macrosomic baby born to a diabetic mother.
Right: A normal baby born to a non-diabetic mother.

Understanding the risks

- Perinatal mortality
- Congenital anomalies
- Maternal mortality
- Diabetic complications in pregnancy
- Obstetric complications
- Inheritance of diabetes in offspring

What a diabetic pregnancy involves

- Frequent antenatal visits and close supervision
- Strict blood glucose control (home blood glucose monitoring, optimized insulin regimen)
- Stop smoking and drinking alcohol
- Appropriate diet

Other advice

- Folic acid supplementation
- Contraception
- Medication

Management of pregnancy in women with diabetes begins with preconception advice and counselling. This includes explanation of the risks of pregnancy, and the requirements for successful pregnancy, including frequent clinic visits beginning as soon as possible after conception, optimized metabolic control, stopping both smoking and drinking alcohol, and a folate-rich and -supplemented diet (5 mg/day – a higher dose than usually recommended for non-diabetic pregnancy). Potentially teratogenic drugs should be replaced with safer alternatives – ACE inhibitors are contraindicated, for example. Outpatient preconception care of diabetic women is thought to reduce congenital anomalies by about two-thirds.

FIGURE 27.4
Prepregnancy counselling.

First trimester management of pregnancy in type 1 diabetes includes optimization of glycaemic control. The strict targets (fasting plasma glucose concentration <5 mmol/L, postprandial peaks <7 mmol/L) virtually always require a basal-bolus insulin injection regimen with four-times daily blood glucose monitoring. Continuous subcutaneous insulin infusion (CSII – insulin pump therapy) is an alternative, especially in those who suffer unacceptable hypoglycaemia (see Chapter 10). Screening for complications is necessary, since pregnancy can worsen renal function in women with established nephropathy; consequently, blood pressure should be tightly controlled (e.g. with nifedipine or methyldopa). Increased proteinuria and hypertension, typical of worsening nephropathy, also occur in pre-eclampsia (see below). Retinopathy, especially preproliferative and proliferative, may also deteriorate rapidly during pregnancy, especially when glycaemic control is suddenly improved; prophylactic photocoagulation should be considered in high-risk patients in early pregnancy or before conception. Myocardial infarction in pregnant diabetic women carries high maternal and fetal mortality; occult ischaemic heart disease should be sought by resting or exercise electrocardiograms.

First trimester

Optimize glycaemic control
- Home blood glucose monitoring
- Education
- Optimize insulin therapy
- Check glycated haemoglobin

Blood glucose targets
- Fasting BG: <5 mmol/L
- Postprandial BG: <7 mmol/L
- HbA_{1c}: normal range

Screen for complications
- Nephropathy (proteinuria, serum creatinine)
- Retinopathy (visual acuity, fundoscopy)
- Vascular disease (BP, ECG)

Diet
- Folate supplements

Discourage smoking and alcohol

Check all medication and discontinue if not essential or if teratogenic

Obstetric assessment
- Ultrasound scan (gestational age, crown–rump length, congenital anomalies, multiple pregnancies, etc.)

FIGURE 27.5
First trimester management of diabetic pregnancy.

HANDBOOK OF DIABETES 3RD EDITION

Obstetric assessment includes regular ultrasound scans to determine gestational age, detecting major malformations, monitoring fetal growth and assessing the volume of the amniotic fluid. The maternal complications of diabetic pregnancy include pre-eclampsia (hypertension, proteinuria, oedema and fetal compromise), polyhydramnios, urinary tract infections, vaginal candidiasis, carpal tunnel syndrome, reflux oesophagitis and preterm labour.

Insulin requirements usually increase gradually through the second trimester, coinciding with increasing insulin resistance and food intake, and may continue to increase until 34–36 weeks' gestation. Serum fructosamine is often considered a useful index of integrated glycaemic control in diabetic pregnancy, where control changes rapidly – it reflects glycaemia over the preceding 2 weeks or so (c.f. HbA$_{1c}$ which measures control over the preceding 6–8 weeks—see Chapter 9). However, it is best to adjust insulin dosages using self-monitored blood glucose tests.

Second trimester

Monitor glycaemic control
- Home blood glucose monitoring
- Increased insulin dosage usual

Increased risk of spontaneous miscarriage if control poor

Monitor and treat complications
- Hypertension: methyldopa, nifedipine
- Retinopathy: photocoagulation

Fetal monitoring
- Ultrasound
  18–22 weeks: major malformations including fetal echocardiography
  26 weeks onwards: growth and liquor volume

Obstetric assessment, check for complications
- Pre-eclampsia
- Polyhydramnios
- Urinary tract infections
- Vaginal candidiasis
- Carpal tunnel syndrome
- Reflux oesophagitis

Third trimester

Monitor glycaemic control
- Insulin dose increases to 34–36 weeks, then plateau and possible small decline

Monitor fetal growth
- Frequent ultrasound scans for accelerated growth (abdominal : head circumference) and liquor volume

Maternal complications
- Pre-eclampsia
- Preterm labour

Plan delivery

FIGURE 27.6
Second and third trimester management of diabetic pregnancy.

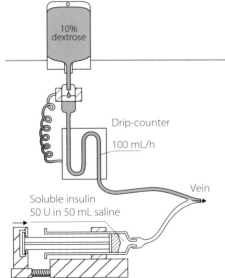

10% dextrose

Drip-counter
100 mL/h

Vein

Soluble insulin
50 U in 50 mL saline

Syringe-driver pump
Titrate rate from hourly blood glucose measurements

During labour, diabetes should be controlled by continuous intravenous infusions of insulin (typically 2–4 units/h) and glucose. After delivery, insulin requirements return rapidly to prepregnancy values and insulin should be reduced to avoid hypoglycaemia. Elective Caesarean section is indicated if mechanical problems with vaginal delivery are anticipated (e.g. malpresentation or disproportion), for fetal compromise and severe pre-eclampsia.

FIGURE 27.7
Intravenous insulin–glucose infusion system for controlling diabetes during labour.

The numbers of pregnant women with type 2 diabetes are increasing, especially in the developing world where this type of diabetes predominates. Women with type 2 diabetes are more likely to present late with pregnancy and to have other risk factors for poor outcome, such as obesity and greater age and parity. Management of pregnancy in type 2 diabetes is the same as that for type 1 diabetes. In general, women should change to insulin before conception or early in the first trimester. Oral hypoglycaemic agents are unlikely to achieve sufficiently good glycaemic control; moreover, some cross the placenta, may aggravate fetal hyperinsulinaemia and are potentially teratogenic (although evidence is conflicting). Glibenclamide (glyburide), however, does not cross the placenta and can be used if insulin treatment is impracticable.

Special features of pregnancy in type 2 diabetes
• In populations where frequency of type 2 diabetes is high (e.g. ethnic minorities), can be more common than pregnancy in type 1 diabetes
• Patients older, more obese than pregnant type 1 diabetic women
• Maternal hypertension more common
• Later presentation
• High rate of fetal loss

FIGURE 27.8
Special features of pregnancy in type 2 diabetes.

Gestational diabetes mellitus (GDM) is glucose intolerance first recognized in pregnancy. It includes previously undiagnosed IGT and type 2 diabetes. No diagnostic criteria are agreed universally, but the World Health Organization definition (which is similar to IGT outside pregnancy, i.e. plasma glucose >7.8 mmol/L 2 hours after a 75 g oral glucose load), is increasingly used. A major trial (HAPO, the Hyperglycaemic Adverse Pregnancy Outcome study) is underway to define the glycaemic thresholds during a 75 g oral glucose tolerance test that are associated with adverse pregnancy outcomes. Risk factors for GDM include obesity, a family history of type 2 diabetes and GDM, a macrosomic infant, unexplained stillbirth or neonatal death during a previous pregnancy, and belonging to a high-risk ethnic group.

Obesity (≥120% ideal bodyweight)
Family history of diabetes
Previous diabetes (associated with oral contraceptive usage or pregnancy)
Previous macrosomic infant, unexplained stillbirth or neonatal death during previous pregnancy
Glycosuria on two or more occasions during current pregnancy
High-risk ethnic group

FIGURE 27.9
Clinical risk factors for gestational diabetes.

Treatment is controversial, but the glycaemic targets should be the same as for established diabetes; about 10–30% of cases require insulin. Diabetes resolves after delivery, but is likely to recur in subsequent pregnancies, and the lifetime risk of developing type 2 diabetes is about 30%. Women who have had GDM therefore need health education about reducing overweight and obesity, increasing exercise and improving their cardiovascular risk profile.

DIABETES IN CHILDHOOD AND ADOLESCENCE

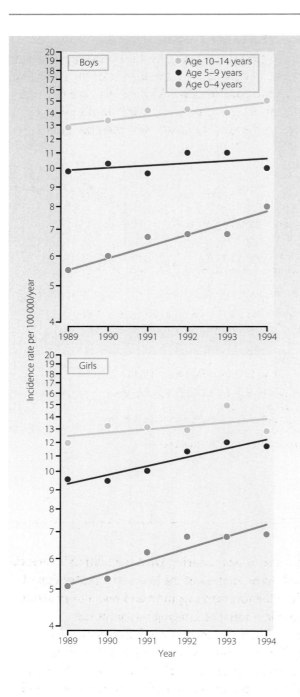

Over 95% of cases of diabetes in children are type 1 diabetes, caused by autoimmune destruction of the islet β cells. The incidence of type 1 diabetes in childhood is increasing, with an average 3% annual increase in Europe and a particularly steep rise in those <5 years of age. This suggests changes in environmental factors that operate early in life. Rarer causes of diabetes in childhood include cystic fibrosis (which usually requires insulin), the rare transient and permanent neonatal forms of diabetes, maturity-onset diabetes of the young (MODY, see Chapter 8) and various other genetic syndromes such as Down's syndrome, Wolfram or DIDMOAD syndrome (diabetes insipidus, diabetes mellitus, optic atrophy and deafness), lipoatrophic diabetes, and diabetes associated with mitochondrial mutations (see Chapter 8). Type 2 diabetes is also increasing in childhood (see below).

FIGURE 28.1

Trends in childhood diabetes incidence in Europe during 1989–1994, by age group and sex.

	Symptom noted n (%)	First symptom noted by the family n (%)
Polyuria	1159 (96%)	854 (71%)
Weight loss	731 (61%)	104 (9%)
Fatigue	630 (52%)	82 (7%)
Abdominal pain	277 (23%)	31 (3%)
Changes in character	137 (11%)	22 (2%)
Others	238 (19%)	36 (3%)
No symptom/unspecified	16 (1%)	78 (6%)

FIGURE 28.2

Symptoms before diagnosis in 1260 children with type 1 diabetes.

Childhood diabetes usually presents acutely with polyuria (including nocturia and incontinence), thirst and polydipsia; about 40% have diabetic ketoacidosis (DKA). Other symptoms are weight loss, fatigue and abdominal pain. A simultaneous febrile illness is noted in about 20% of cases, particularly in younger children. Other possible presenting features include muscle cramps, infections (e.g. boils, urinary tract infections), behaviour disturbance and poor school performance.

As with adults, DKA in children is a medical emergency that requires urgent admission to hospital, intravenous rehydration and insulin infusion. Saline (0.9%) should be given intravenously at a rate of 8–10 mL/kg over the first hour, depending on the severity of dehydration and the age of the child (less in those <5 years of age). Unless there is initial hyperkalaemia, potassium is added early, at the rate of 20 mmol/L of saline. The usual rate of insulin infusion is 0.1 units/kg/h or 0.05 units/kg/h in the child <5 years of age. The initial saline infusion should be replaced by 5% glucose (dextrose) when the plasma glucose reaches about 14 mmol/L.

Parameters	Clinical and biological assessment	Treatment
Conscious level	Clinical exam: Glasgow Coma Score, calculated osmolality	Consider ICU, airway protection, nasogastric intubation, urinary catheterization
Hydration status	Shock Heart rate, blood pressure Sodium, urea, creatinine Urine output	• Consider macromolecule Plasmion 20 mL/kg in 20 min • IV access: normal saline 10 mL/kg/h or 8 mL/kg/h in the child < 5 years • No more than 2 h, then change to glucose
Insulin deficiency	Respiratory pattern Venous pH and bicarbonate, fall in plasma glucose Ketonuria, anion gap	IV insulin infusion (no bolus): 0.1 units/kg/h, except 0.05/kg/h in the child < 5 years, then adapt insulin infusion rate to
Potassium status	Plasma K+, ECG	Add KCl to IV fluid (20 mmol/L of intravenous fluid)
Plasma glucose	Hourly bedside	• 5% glucose, then 10% glucose when plasma glucose < 14 mmol/L, at 3 L/m2/24 h. • Adjust insulin to obtain a fall in plasma glucose of no more than 5 mmol/L/h • No more than 4 L/m2/day of fluid altogether

FIGURE 28.3
Suggested treatment for diabetic ketoacidosis in children.

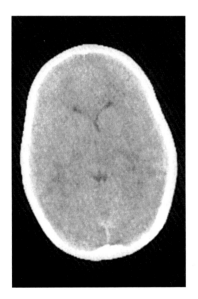

The most common cause of death during DKA in children is cerebral oedema, which leads to herniation of the brain stem, extension of the cerebellar tonsils into the foramen magnum and respiratory arrest. It is diagnosed by magnetic resonance imaging or computed tomography of the brain. Clinically, there is headache, depressed consciousness (falling Glasgow Coma Scale score) and sometimes papilloedema. Risk factors include low arterial PCO_2, elevated blood urea and treatment with bicarbonate. Over-rapid delivery of fluid and insulin may also be involved. The treatment involves intravenous mannitol (20% mannitol, 2.5 mL/kg over 15 minutes, repeated if necessary). See Chapter 12 for further details of DKA.

FIGURE 28.4
CT scan of the brain of a child with diabetic ketoacidosis complicated by cerebral oedema. There is marked swelling of the brain substance with compression of the lateral ventricles.

Twice-daily injections of short- and intermediate-acting insulins are most common in paediatric practice, including premixed formulations and the use of insulin 'pens'. Monomeric insulins, such as lispro or aspart, which can be injected with or even after meals, are helpful in toddlers with their erratic appetites. These analogues may also reduce nocturnal hypoglycaemia. After the diagnosis of diabetes, there is sometimes a partial remission (the 'honeymoon period'), lasting from a few months to 2 years, during which the insulin dose is <0.5 units/kg. This is due to a transient improvement in residual β-cell function. It is usual to maintain low-dose insulin treatment during the honeymoon period.

Hypoglycaemia is common in diabetic children, particularly in younger children, who cannot communicate and in whom signs of hypoglycaemia (pallor, drowsiness, lethargy) are often detected by the parents. Moreover, young children are at risk of later neuropsychological impairment from severe, recurrent hypoglycaemia. Presumably, this relates to the effect of hypoglycaemia on the developing brain. Even older children are less able to detect hypoglycaemia than adults. Behavioural manifestations of hypoglycaemia include aggression, irritability, sadness, fatigue and naughtiness.

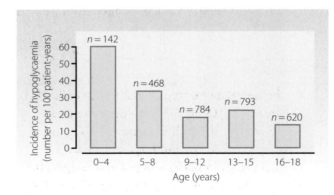

FIGURE 28.5
Incidence of hypoglycaemia (unconsciousness or seizures) in different age groups with type 1 diabetes.

Neuroglycopenic and autonomic	Behavioural
Reported by the children	
Weakness	Headache
Trembling	Argumentative
Dizziness	Aggressive
Poor concentration	Irritability
Hunger	Naughty
Sweating	
Confusion	
Blurred vision	
Slurred speech	Nausea
Double vision	Nightmares
Observed by the parents	
As above, plus:	
Pallor	
Sleepiness	
Convulsions	

FIGURE 28.6
Clinical features of hypoglycaemia in children.

Continuous subcutaneous insulin infusion (CSII, insulin pump therapy) is an alternative option for achieving strict metabolic control in selected patients, particularly in children who have been unable to maintain good control with multiple-dose injection therapy, without frequent, unpredictable and disabling hypoglycaemia. Experience of CSII in children is less extensive than that in adults and, although rapidly gaining in popularity, more long-term study is needed. As with adults, careful selection of patients and a healthcare team experienced in insulin pump therapy are essential (see Chapter 10).

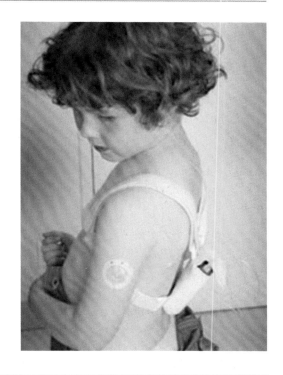

FIGURE 28.7
Insulin pump treatment of a child with type 1 diabetes.

Diabetic control often deteriorates in adolescence, particularly in girls. The reasons for this include both metabolic factors, especially the normal insulin resistance of puberty, and psychological problems caused by the interference of diabetes with the normal increasing independence from parents during adolescence.

Features suggestive of type 2 diabetes

Family history of type 2 diabetes

High-risk ethnic groups: African-American, Asian, Caribbean, Hispanic

Obesity

Female sex

Pubertal period

Clinical signs of insulin resistance: acanthosis nigricans, polycystic ovary signs

Biological signs of insulin resistance: detectable, high or normal insulin or C-peptide level

No insulin therapy necessary for survival

Negative facts in favour of type 2 diabetes

No HLA haplotypes associated with type 1 diabetes

No signs of autoimmunity: no anti-islet cell antibodies

The prevalence of type 2 diabetes in children is increasing in parallel with the increase in childhood obesity. When diabetes is diagnosed, most are undergoing puberty, so perhaps the normal insulin resistance of puberty triggers the diabetes. Most also belong to a high-risk ethnic group – of African, Caribbean, Asian or Hispanic descent. There are usually clinical signs of insulin resistance, such as acanthosis nigricans or the polycystic ovary syndrome. The pathophysiology of type 2 diabetes in childhood is probably similar to that in adults (see Chapter 7).

FIGURE 28.8
Diagnostic criteria for type 2 diabetes in children.

247

Diabetes and impaired glucose tolerance are common in elderly people, each of which affects about 10–30% of subjects over the age of 65 years in many Western countries. There are particularly high frequencies in certain susceptible ethnic groups, such as Black Americans and Mexican Americans (about 30% of the elderly). Type 2 diabetes accounts for about 95% of cases of diabetes in old age in most populations and virtually all in ethnic minorities.

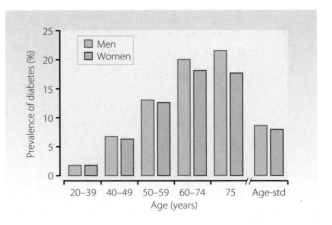

FIGURE 29.1
Prevalence of diabetes in men and women in the US population of age ≥20 years, based on the NHANES III study. Subjects include those with previously diagnosed and undiagnosed diabetes (defined by fasting plasma glucose ≥7.0 mmol/L). Age-std, age-standardized.

The presentation of diabetes in older people is often insidious and its diagnosis delayed. Symptoms can be non-specific and vague, such as fatigue, urinary incontinence or change in mental state (e.g. depression, confusion and apathy). Many cases are detected by finding hyperglycaemia during the investigation of comorbidities, such as a delayed recovery from intercurrent illnesses, repeated infections or cardiovascular disease; the latter may present with atypical features, such as painless myocardial infarction, manifested as breathlessness, lassitude or falls. Lower-limb ischaemia can occur without claudication, and even presents first with gangrene. Worryingly, even when coincidental hyperglycaemia is recognized in hospital, many elderly people receive no further evaluation or treatment.

Acute metabolic disturbance is rarer: ~25% of cases of hyperosmolar non-ketotic hyperglycaemic coma (HONK, see Chapter 12) occur in people with previously undiagnosed type 2 diabetes. HONK predominantly affects those older than 50 years of age. The tendency to hyperosmolarity may be worse in elderly people, who may not perceive thirst or drink enough to compensate for the osmotic diuresis of diabetes, and who are often taking diuretics. Rarely, diabetic ketoacidosis is the presenting feature of type 1 diabetes in the elderly.

- Non-specific symptoms
  (lassitude, confusion, incontinence, falls, etc.)

- Presentation with comorbidity (coincidental hyperglycaemia)

  - cardiovascular disease
    (NB myocardial infarction may be silent in the elderly)

  - delayed recovery from illness (e.g. stroke)

  - repeated infections

- Classic osmotic symptoms1

- Acute metabolic disturbance (mostly HONK, rarely DKA)

FIGURE 29.2
Modes of presentation of diabetes in the elderly.

HANDBOOK OF DIABETES 3RD EDITION

Elderly diabetic people require treatment mainly to alleviate symptoms, to reduce the risk of hyperglycaemic crises, to prevent and manage vascular and other complications and to achieve a normal life expectancy whenever possible. Strict glycaemic control may not always be appropriate. Diets rarely produce weight loss in the elderly and may be unjustifiably burdensome in the frail. Short-acting sulphonylureas such as gliclazide and tolbutamide, are preferred because of the likelihood in the elderly of impaired renal function, poor nutrition, impaired counter-regulatory responses and cognition, and other factors that increase the risk of hypoglycaemia. Metformin is best avoided in many elderly subjects because of its increased tendency to cause lactic acidosis with renal impairment and hepatic or cardiac failure.

General hazards of drug treatment in the elderly include the possibility of multiple drug interactions, non-compliance and inappropriate drug prescribing.

Diabetes in the elderly

- Diet often unsuccessful
- Use short-acting sulphonylureas
- Avoid metformin
- Use simple insulin regimens
- Note drug hazards in the elderly

FIGURE 29.3
Diabetes in the elderly: treatment points.

Simple insulin regimens are usually the most appropriate in diabetes of old age. Twice-daily injections of premixed insulins for type 1 diabetes or isophane in type 2 patients are preferred. However, the practical difficulties of administration can limit their use in some patients and once-daily insulin, though unlikely to produce good control, may be more suitable for the very old and frail. The use of once- or twice-daily injections of the new long-acting insulin analogue glargine may be advantageous and needs to be explored in elderly diabetic subjects. A multiple-dose, basal-bolus regimen can achieve near normoglycaemia, but is probably only suitable for the comparatively few well-motivated, mobile and mentally alert patients who are independent in self-care and have no other major medical disorders.

	Indications	Advantages	Disadvantages
Once-daily insulin	• Frail subjects • Very old (> 80 y) • Symptomatic control	• Single injection • Can be given by carer or district nurse	• Control usually poor • Hypoglycaemia common
Twice-daily insulin	• Preferred if good glycaemic control • Suitable for type 1 diabetes	• Low risk of hypoglycaemia • Easily managed by most older diabetic people • Expensive	• Normoglycaemia difficult to achieve • Fixed meal times reduce flexibility
Basal/bolus insulin	• Well-motivated individuals • Can reduce microvascular complications	• Enables tight control • For acute illness in hospital • Flexible meal times	• Frequent monitoring required to avoid hypoglycaemia
Insulin plus oral agents	• If glycaemic control is unsatisfactory with oral agents alone • To limit weight gain in obese subjects	• Limits weight gain by reducing total daily insulin • Increased flexibility	• May delay conversion to insulin in thin or type 1 patients

FIGURE 29.4
General guidelines for treatment in older people.

DIABETES AND LIFESTYLE   30

- Newly diagnosed patients, especially insulin-treated, should not drive until glycaemic control and vision are stable
- Recurrent daytime hypoglycaemia, particularly if severe
- Impaired awareness of hypoglycaemia, if disabling
- Reduced visual acuity in both eyes (i.e. worse than 6/12 on Snellen chart)
- Severe sensorimotor peripheral neuropathy, especially with loss of proprioception
- Severe peripheral vascular disease
- Lower limb amputation

FIGURE 30.1
Reasons for diabetic drivers to stop driving.

Driving

In many countries, drivers with diabetes are legally required to declare the diagnosis to the national licensing authority and to the vehicle insurer. The main problems for diabetic drivers are hypoglycaemia and visual impairment from cataract or retinopathy. Rarely, disability from severe neuropathy, peripheral vascular disease or leg amputation can present mechanical difficulties, but usually these can be overcome by adapting the vehicle or using automatic transmission. Despite these problems, the overall accident rate for diabetic subjects appears to be no higher than that for non-diabetic people.

General advice to the diabetic driver includes the requirements in most countries to declare diabetes to the relevant authorities. Diabetic drivers must actively avoid hypoglycaemia – motor skills and judgement can be reduced at blood glucose levels of 3–4 mmol/L (54–72 mg/dL), without obvious hypoglycaemic symptoms. Impaired awareness of hypoglycaemia is therefore a relative contraindication to driving. If hypoglycaemia occurs while driving, subjects should stop, leave the driver's seat and wait 45–60 minutes before driving again. Hypoglycaemia can resemble alcohol intoxication and diabetic people can be arrested on the assumption that they are drunk – they should therefore carry an identity card or bracelet that states they have diabetes.

- Inform licensing authority (statutory requirement) and motor insurer of diabetes and its treatment
- Do not drive if eyesight deteriorates suddenly
- Check blood glucose before driving (even on short journeys) and at intervals on longer journeys
- Take frequent rests with snacks or meals; avoid alcohol
- Keep a supply of fast- and longer-acting carbohydrate in the vehicle for emergency use
- Carry personal identification to indicate that you have diabetes (and are prone to hypoglycaemia)
- If hypoglycaemia develops, stop driving, switch off engine, leave the driver's seat and then treat the episode
- Do not resume driving for 60 min after blood glucose has returned to normal

FIGURE 30.2
Advice for diabetic drivers.

Corrected visual acuity worse than about 6/12 in the better eye precludes driving in the general population in many countries (e.g. in the UK), but diabetic subjects with better acuity than this may still have visual field loss, poor night vision and impaired perception of movement because of retinopathy, laser treatment or cataracts.

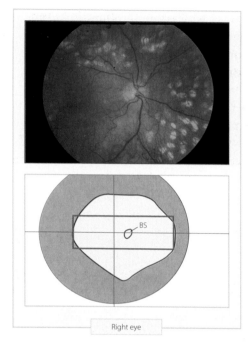

Right eye

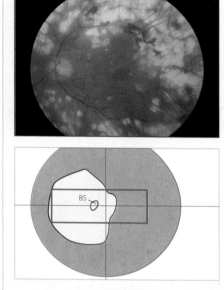

Left eye

FIGURE 30.3
Visual field loss due to photocoagulation. This 60-year-old diabetic man needed heavy laser photocoagulation to the temporal retina of the left eye, which caused nasal visual field loss such that this eye failed the standard test for driving. The right eye required less intensive laser treatment and the visual field was adequate for driving. He was allowed to drive. BS, blind spot. Blue rectangle: minimum area recommended for safe driving.

Vocational (professional) driving
Large goods vehicles (LGV)
Passenger-carrying vehicles (PCV)
Locomotives and underground trains
Professional drivers (chauffeurs)
Taxi drivers (variable; depends on local authority)

National and emergency services
Armed forces (army, navy, air force)
Police force
Fire brigade or rescue services
Merchant navy
Prison and security services

Civil aviation
Commercial pilots and flight engineers
Aircrew
Air-traffic controllers

Dangerous working areas
Offshore: oil rigs, gas platforms
Moving machinery
Incinerators and hot-metal areas
Work on railway tracks
Coal mining
Heights: overhead lines, cranes, scaffolding

Employment

Diabetic people can and should be encouraged to undertake a wide range of employment. Employment is generally restricted where hypoglycaemia poses a risk to the diabetic worker or to his or her colleagues. In most countries, employment is disbarred in the armed forces, civil aviation, emergency services such as fire fighting, in many forms of commercial driving and in dangerous areas such as off-shore and overhead working. Sometimes restrictions have been established by particular firms or industries, rather than by legislation. Individual assessment is desirable to take account of the type and method of treatment of diabetes.

FIGURE 30.4
Forms of employment from which insulin-treated diabetic people are generally excluded in the UK.

Smoking

Smoking is one of the major avoidable causes of ill health and death. Smoking is a powerful independent risk factor for macrovascular disease and enhances the cardiovascular risk and mortality associated with diabetes. Smoking is also a risk factor for the development of type 2 diabetes, may predispose to microvascular and other complications and is associated with poorer glycaemic control. Strenuous efforts should be made to discourage smoking in diabetic patients, but anti-smoking policies often fail. Fear of weight gain is a common reason for not giving up smoking. Measures to aid cessation of smoking include special 'stop-smoking clinics', nicotine replacement (chewing gum or nasal sprays are probably better than dermal patches) and oral bupropion (a catecholamine reuptake inhibitor that may reduce craving and withdrawal symptoms; it can provoke seizures and is therefore contraindicated in those at risk of severe hypoglycaemia). Results of all these measures can be disappointing.

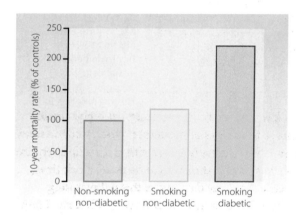

FIGURE 30.5
Deleterious effects of smoking and disease on 10-year mortality. Death rate is expressed as a percentage of that in age- and sex-matched non-diabetic, non-smoking populations.

Potentially diabetogenic
- Impairs glucose tolerance and insulin sensitivity
- Independent risk factor for type 2 diabetes

Atherogenic
- Independent risk factor: enhances atherogenic effect of diabetes
- Coagulation and haemorheological changes (increase viscosity, fibrinogen, free radicals and endothelial damage)

Risk factor for diabetic complications
- Retinopathy
- Nephropathy
- Limited joint mobility and necrobiosis lipoidica

Increases mortality

FIGURE 30.6
Suggested deleterious effects of smoking in diabetes.

Travel

Diabetes is not a bar to travelling, but planning is needed for extra supplies, insurance, medical identification, and changes in meals, fluid intake, physical activity and antidiabetic treatment *en route* and after arrival.

Documents
Diabetes identity card or bracelet
Document stating diagnosis and treatment
Blood glucose monitoring diary
Equipment
Insulin vials or cartridges
Syringes and needles (or pens and spare pen needles)
Flask or cool bag for insulin storage
Blood glucose meter; spare meter and batteries
Finger pricker and spare lancets; container for used needles
Blood glucose test-strips (visual reading)
Fluids
Glucose-free drinks (screw-top container)
Bottled water (plastic container)
Hypoglycaemia treatment
Quick-acting carbohydrate
• Glucose drinks (screw-top container)
• Glucose tablets/confectionery
Slow-acting carbohydrate
• Biscuits or cereal bars

FIGURE 30.7
Checklist of essential items for travellers with insulin-treated diabetes.

During long flights, blood glucose should be monitored frequently (every 2–3 hours) and glycaemic control may need to be relaxed to avoid hypoglycaemia: a few hours of moderate hyperglycaemia, say 10–13 mmol/L (180–234 mg/dL), is acceptable. Time changes of less than 4 hours in either direction require no major adjustments to the usual insulin schedule – simply give the next insulin at its usual clock time, using the destination's time zone. Westward flights effectively extend the day, and if this delay is long (>6–8 hours), extra insulin may be needed – small doses of rapid-acting insulin injected 3–4 hourly. Long-acting insulin doses before eastward flights, which shorten the day, may need to be reduced if shortened by >6–8 hours.

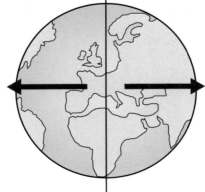

Flying West:
'day' is lengthened

• Pre-flight:
give normal doses

• In-flight:
may need additional insulin if day lengthened by >8 h

• Post-flight:
give next dose at usual clock-time (new time-zone)

Flying East:
'day' is shortened

• Pre-flight:
reduce dose if day will be shortened by >8 h

• In-flight:
monitor glucose

• Post-flight:
give next dose at usual clock time (new time-zone)

Always:
• Monitor blood glucose 2–3 hourly
• Relax glycaemic control (8–13 mmol/L)
• Use small doses of soluble insulin or rapid-acting analogue to treat hyperglycaemia
• Treat hypoglycaemia promptly

FIGURE 30.8
Scheme for adjusting insulin dosages during flights that cross time zones.

ORGANIZATION OF DIABETES CARE: DIABETES SPECIALIST NURSING, DIABETES EDUCATION AND GENERAL PRACTICE

31

N̲o single person can provide all that is required in diabetes care. Modern management consists of an interacting team that involves many hospital specialists (e.g. physicians, ophthalmologists, paediatricians, psychologists, nephrologists, obstetricians, specialist nurses, dietitians, chiropodists, etc.), general practitioners and their team, diabetes associations, government departments and, most importantly, the patient and his or her family and friends.

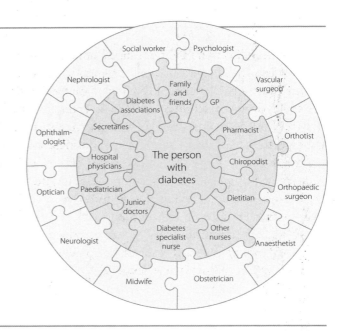

FIGURE 31.1
The diabetes care team and how it fits together.

D̲iabetes specialist nurses play a crucial role in diabetes care, with important duties in clinical care and advice, education of patients and healthcare professionals, counselling and helping to implement lifestyle changes in diabetic patients.

FIGURE 31.2
The multifaceted roles of the diabetes specialist nurse.

D̲iabetes education programmes, which are usually run by diabetes specialist nurses, have been shown to improve major diabetes outcomes, such as time spent in hospital or off work and the rate of amputations.

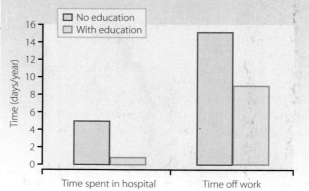

FIGURE 31.3
Effects of diabetes education on hospitalization and ability to work.

Diabetes education methods range from one-to-one meetings, through group sessions with other patients, to computer-based learning. Interaction and questioning should be encouraged; didactic lectures generally fail to alter behaviour. Counselling skills are important in helping patients to cope with the anger, denial or depression that may accompany the diagnosis of diabetes. Clear objectives should be drawn up for education and agreed with each patient. Children, adolescents and elderly people are among the diabetic groups that require special consideration in education schemes because of problems with compliance, adjusting their lifestyle, speed of learning, and ability and willingness to assume responsibility for their own care. Lack of time often makes it difficult to provide adequate education for diabetic people; accordingly, the Diabetes Education Study Group (DESG) of the European Association for the Study of Diabetes has produced brief 'Teaching Letters' for healthcare professionals, a '5-Minute Survival Kit' and a list of 'Patient Education Basics'. These have been translated into 27 languages and can be downloaded from the DESG website (www.desg.org).

1 Oral agents
2 Hypoglycaemia
3 Self-monitoring
4 Putting a patient on a diet
5 Counselling on late complications
6 Foot care
7 Patient education: a lifelong process
8 Therapeutics and education (with poster)
9 Help your patients to improve self-management: building a therapeutic chain (poster)
10 Managing the patient with excess weight and diabetes
11 Checklist for diabetic patient education
12 How to improve follow-up in long-term disease
13 Motivating the diabetic patient
14 My patient is poorly controlled: how do I approach this problem?
15 Right from the start: education at the time of diagnosis
16 Diabetic retinopathy and therapeutic education
17 Educational approach to the elderly diabetic patient
18 Group versus individual therapeutic patient education
19 Therapeutic diabetes education in camp settings
20 The function of psychosocial support in diabetes education
21 Therapeutic education: what a diabetes centre should provide
22 Planning an educational program
23 Diabetes education and cost control: time to measure
24 Evaluating diabetes education

FIGURE 31.4
'Teaching Letters' published by the Diabetes Education Study Group of the European Association for the Study of Diabetes (see www.desg.org).

1 Prevention of hypoglycaemia; initiating insulin treatment
2 Intercurrent illness, sick-day rules and acetone
3 Meal planning: type 1 diabetes
4 Meal planning: type 2 diabetes
5 Weight loss: type 2 diabetes
6 Prevention of foot lesions. For patients with no vascular or neuropathic problems
7 Loss of pain sensation. Long-term complications and prevention of amputations
8 Follow-up of eye problems
9 Pregnancy and diabetes

FIGURE 31.5
The 5-Minute Survival Kit. From the Diabetes Education Study Group of the European Association for the Study of Diabetes (see www.desg.org).

1 How to prevent low blood sugar
2 Lose weight by eating better
3 Diabetic retinopathy and follow-up of eye problems
4 Prevention of foot problems
5 You have type 2 diabetes'—meaning and implications
6 Preventing late diabetic complications
7 Ageing and diabetes management
8 Improving follow-up in long-term disease
9 Blood-glucose monitoring: a must in diabetes management
10 Diabetes treatment and 'others' (the role of the family and the social environment)
11 Prevention of heart problems
12 Physical exercise: a therapy for diabetes at all ages
13 Intercurrent diseases: a challenge for diabetes control
14 Preventing diabetes in your relatives

FIGURE 31.6
List of patient education basics for type 2 diabetes. From the Diabetes Education Study Group of the European Association for the Study of Diabetes.

Shared care between hospital and general practice is the most realistic way to ensure optimal management of diabetic people. Primary care can provide early contact with the patient, and therefore opportunities to screen, diagnose and prevent complications. General practitioners can also offer long-term medical, psychological, social and family support needed for chronic multisystem diseases such as diabetes.

Some of the essential elements of hospital and general practice care include:
- an agreed check-list and guidelines for procedures to be performed;
- agreed sharing of responsibilities and mechanism of exchange of information;
- a substantial structure, adequate support and appropriate training for care in general practice; and
- centrally computerized prompted recall and review of patients.

	At diagnosis	Routine visits, approx. every 3 months	Annual reviews
Review patients' perceived problems	✓	✓	✓
Discuss patients' diabetes diary, home measurements (blood glucose, blood pressure) and history of hypo- or hyperglycaemic symptoms		✓	✓
A complete objective examination	✓		
Objective examination according to needs		✓	✓
Height	✓		
Weight	✓	✓	✓
Blood pressure	✓	✓	✓
Electrocardiogram	✓		✓
Blood glucose and HbA1c	✓	✓	✓
Lipids	✓	✓	✓
Creatinine and electrolytes	✓		✓
Urine for microscopy and culture	✓		✓
Urine albumin/creatinine ratio and ketones	✓	✓	✓
Foot examination, including pulses, hyperkeratosis and examination for neuropathy	✓		✓
Visual acuity, retinal photography or referral to ophthalmologist	✓	✓	✓
Initiation of or follow-up on education needs	✓	✓	✓
Agree on targets for the coming year (lifestyle changes and levels for blood glucose, lipids and blood pressure)	✓		✓
Adjustment of treatment or targets according to effects and side-effects		✓	✓
Consider special needs and problems related to society, work or family, including exploration of sexual problems, need for contraception or hormone-replacement therapy	✓		✓
Consider need for referral to chiropodist, diabetic nurse or dietitian	✓	✓	✓
Inspection of injection sites			✓
Check of self-monitoring technique and device, i.e. blood glucose and/or blood pressure device			✓
Agreement on next visit	✓	✓	✓

FIGURE 31.7
Proposal for checklist at diagnosis, routine visits and annual reviews.

FUTURE DIRECTIONS IN DIABETES MANAGEMENT AND RESEARCH

Pancreas and islet-cell transplantation

Until recent advances in islet-cell transplantation, whole or segmental pancreas transplantation was the only treatment for type 1 diabetes able to restore endogenous insulin secretion. Currently, about 1500 whole-pancreas transplants take place every year, worldwide. Functioning graft survival is generally better with simultaneous pancreas–kidney grafts than with a pancreas-alone transplant.

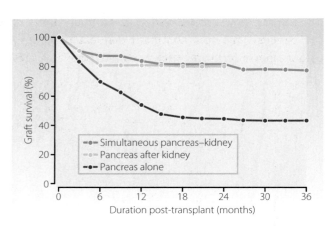

FIGURE 32.1
Pancreas-alone graft survival is inferior to pancreas–kidney transplantation.

Recent advances that have improved the outcome of whole-pancreas transplantation are enteric exocrine drainage by graft duodenojejunal anastomosis (rather than drainage into the bladder), primary portal vein drainage (rather than into the systemic circulation) and better and safer immunosuppression with tacrolimus and mycophenolate. The progression of diabetic complications can be halted or reversed by pancreas transplantation if there is a sufficient period of post-transplant normoglycaemia – up to 10 years in some cases.

Pancreas

FIGURE 32.2
Portal-enteric pancreas grafts (shown here) have less rejection and improved outcome.

- Type 1 DM, islet-alone, non-HLA match, –ve PRA
- ABO-compatible, sequential transplant, 'double-donor'
- Immediate infusion, percutaneous portal access
- Steroid-free, low-dose calcineurin inhibitor, potent immunosuppression
- Refined isolation protocol—perfusion, Liberase, continuous gradient Ficoll
- No culture, no xenoproteins, no cryopreservation

The clinical outcome for islet-cell transplantation was transformed from the year 2000, with the introduction of the 'Edmonton Protocol' (named after the group at the University of Edmonton, who originated the method). The protocol is based on transplanting an adequate mass of freshly isolated islet cells, providing a potent, steroid-free and less diabetogenic immunosuppression regimen, and careful selection of patients without renal failure. The immunosuppression involves pre- and post-transplant daclizumab (anti-interleukin 2 receptor monoclonal antibody), maintenance sirolimus and low-dose tacrolimus. With this regimen, 100% of the initial type 1 diabetic group treated became insulin-independent.

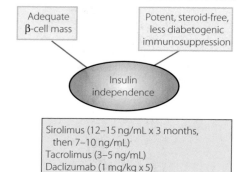

FIGURE 32.3
The 'Edmonton Protocol'. PRA, patient-reactive antibodies; ABO, blood group; HLA, human leukocyte antigen.

The procedure for islet isolation is labour intensive and involves enzymatic fragmentation of the pancreas in a semi-automatic dissociation chamber. Islets are injected or infused percutaneously into the portal vein and embolize into the liver. Two sequential donors are usually used – providing ~850 000 islet equivalents per recipient. Of 32 consecutive type 1 diabetic patients treated in Edmonton, 85% showed sustained insulin-independence and had returned to normoglycaemia at 1 year.

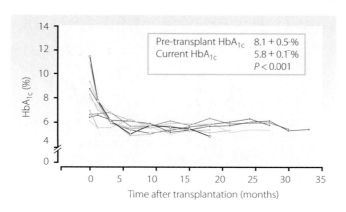

Pre-transplant HbA$_{1c}$ 8.1 + 0.5 %
Current HbA$_{1c}$ 5.8 + 0.1 %
$P < 0.001$

FIGURE 32.4
HbA$_{1c}$ is corrected by successful islet transplantation. Individual patients.

Stem-cell therapy

The aim of stem-cell research in diabetes is to provide a source of cells nearly identical to the pancreatic β cell for treatment of type 1 diabetes by transplantation. Stem cells are self-renewing cells that produce large numbers of differentiated progeny; the two main categories are embryonic and adult stem cells. Embryonic stem cells are derived from the inner cell mass of mammalian blastocysts; they can be cultured *in vitro* and when allowed to aggregate (as an 'embryoid body') they can differentiate into all of the tissues of the embryo, including β cells. The signals that guide embryonic stem cells into endoderm and β cells are largely unknown and strategies have therefore so far included *in vitro* culture and spontaneous differentiation of stem cells with subsequent selection of any cells that express insulin. The similarity of these cells to mature β cells is unclear.

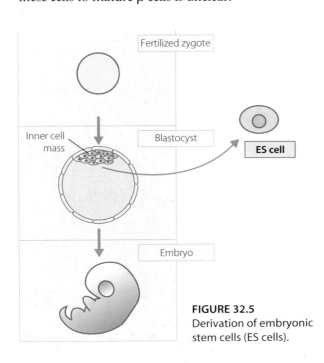

FIGURE 32.5
Derivation of embryonic stem cells (ES cells).

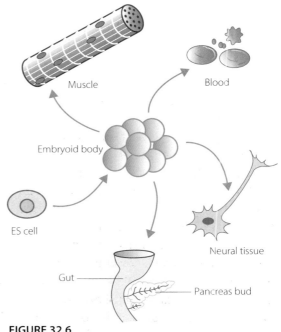

FIGURE 32.6
The pluripotent nature of embryonic stem (ES) cells.

Adult stem cells are thought to be rare, but have been identified in many organs where they participate in tissue repair and homeostasis, notably the bone marrow. Though once thought to be specific for a single organ, they may be able to generate differentiated cells of other organs (e.g. bone-marrow cells that produce liver, muscle or brain cells). The evidence for pancreatic stem cells is largely indirect; for example, after injury to the pancreas in experimental animal studies, new islet cells appear to bud from the ducts and may originate from stem cells at this site (the exact cell population has not been identified).

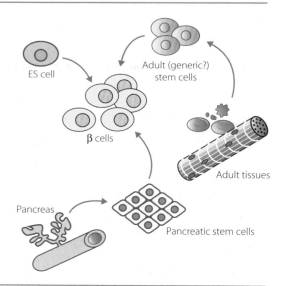

FIGURE 32.7
Potential stem-cell sources of β cells.

Gene therapy

Gene therapy for diabetes is still at the stage of animal experimentation, but the aim is to transfer DNA to somatic cells to treat or prevent diabetes or its complications. Several strategies are envisaged, including prevention of β-cell destruction by manipulating β cells to produce a survival factor (e.g. interleukin-1 receptor antagonist or anti-apoptotic factors). This requires a (currently undescribed) vector to transform the remaining β cells *in vivo* in newly diagnosed type 1 diabetic patients. Immunomodulation might be achieved by DNA vaccination in high-risk individuals, for example using glutamic acid decarboxylase (GAD) DNA to induce tolerance to this key autoantigen. Stimulation of β-cell differentiation and regeneration might involve gene therapy with transcription factors that control development (e.g. Pdx-1). Ectopic production of insulin by several substitute cells has already been achieved, including fibroblasts, hepatocytes and pituitary cells, with glucose responsiveness achieved by placing the insulin gene under the control of glucose-sensitive gene transcription (e.g. glucose-6-phosphatase). K cells from the gut have the same glucose sensor as the β cell and might also be a good substitute cell. Finally, conditionally transformed β cell lines may produce cells in quantity for transplantation.

Strategy	Target cell	Gene product	Desired effect
β-cell protection factor	β cell	IL-1	β-cell survival
DNA vaccination	Muscle	GAD epitope Fas ligand epitope	Immunotolerance
β-cell differentiation and proliferation	β cell/β-cell precursor	Pdx-1	Increased β-cell mass
Insulin production by substitute cells	Hepatocyte K cell Fibroblast Hepatocyte	Insulin/insulin analogue with G6P/PK-promoter Insulin gene with GIP-promoter Insulin/CAD-fusion protein Pdx-1	Glucose-sensitive insulin gene transcription Glucose-sensitive insulin release Oral drug-induced insulin release Hepatocyte transdifferentiation
Conditionally transformed β-cell lines	β cell	Oncogene	To generate β cells for transplantation purposes

FIGURE 32.8
Examples of gene therapy based strategies for treatment or prevention of diabetes mellitus.

ACKNOWLEDGEMENTS

Contributors to the *Textbook of Diabetes,* third edition

Erica L.T. van den Akker, Rotterdam, The Netherlands

John Ayuk, Birmingham, UK

Clifford J. Bailey, Birmingham, UK

Stephen C. Bain, Birmingham, UK

Beverley Balkau, Villejuif, France

Anthony H. Barnett, Birmingham, UK

Christopher Beith, Manchester, UK

Chen Bing, Liverpool, UK

Anne E. Bishop, London, UK

Donatella Bloise, Rome, Italy

Geremia B. Bolli, Perugia, Italy

Adrian J. Bone, Brighton, UK

Knut Borch-Johnsen, Gentofte, Denmark

Michael Brownlee, New York, USA

G. Jan Bruining, Rotterdam, The Netherlands

José Catalan, London, UK

Clive S. Cockram, Shatin, Hong Kong

Kennedy Cruickshank, Manchester, UK

Paul Czernichow, Paris, France

J. Andrew Davies, Leeds, UK

Jean-Pierre Després, Québec, Canada

Julian E. Donckier, Namur, Belgium

Anne Dornhorst, London, UK

Eveline Eschwège, Villejuif, France

Christine Feinle, Adelaide, Australia

Robin E. Ferner, Birmingham, UK

Peter R. Flatt, Coleraine, UK

John V. Forrester, Aberdeen, UK

Brian M. Frier, Edinburgh, UK

Philippe Froguel, Lille, France

Stella George, Cambridge, UK

John E. Gerich, New York, USA

Geoffrey V. Gill, Liverpool, UK

Raj S. Gill, Southampton, UK

Joanna Girling, Middlesex, UK

Neil J.L. Gittoes, Birmingham, UK

Luigi Gnudi, London, UK

Alain Golay, Geneva, Switzerland

Peter J. Grant, Leeds, UK

Lucinda Green, London, UK

Gabriella Gruden, London, UK

Joanne A. Harrold, Liverpool, UK

Andrew T. Hattersley, Exeter, UK

Lutz Heinemann, Neuss, Germany

Simon R. Heller, Sheffield, UK

U. Freddie J. Henriksson, Stockholm, Sweden

Michael Horowitz, Adelaide, Australia

Simon L. Howell, London, UK

Frank B. Hu, Boston, MA, USA

Karen L. Jones, Adelaide, Australia

Bengt Jönsson, Stockholm, Sweden

Nirmal Joshi, Hershey, PA, USA

Hee-Sook Jun, Calgary, Canada

Marjatta Karvonen, Helsinki, Finland

Nicholas Katsilambros, Athens, Greece

M. Ann Kelly, Birmingham, UK

Martin J. Kendall, Birmingham, UK

Glen P. Kenny, Ottawa, Canada

Rachel M. Knott, Aberdeen, UK

Veikko A. Koivisto, Hamburg, Germany

Andrew J. Krentz, Southampton, UK

Yolanta T. Kruszynska, La Jolla, CA, USA

Jonathan R.T. Lakey, Edmonton, Canada

Frank Lally, Birmingham, UK

Torsten Lauritzen, Aarhus, Denmark

R. David G. Leslie, London, UK

Susan Lightman, London, UK

Peter Lindgren, Stockholm, Sweden

Amanda J. MacFarlane, Ottawa, Canada

Monica Mahajan, New Delhi, India

Aldo Maldonato, Rome, Italy

JoAnn E. Manson, Boston, MA, USA

Sally M. Marshall, Newcastle upon Tyne, UK

David R. Matthews, Oxford, UK

Jean Claude N. Mbanya, Yaounde, Cameroon

Douglas A. Melton, Cambridge, MA, USA

Catherine H. Mijovic, Birmingham, UK

V. Mohan, Chennai, India

Malcolm Nattrass, Birmingham, UK

Peter M. Nilsson, Malmö, Sweden

Deirdre O'Donovan, Adelaide, Australia

Stephen O'Rahilly, Cambridge, UK

Badal Pal, West Didsbury, Manchester, UK

Breay W. Paty, Edmonton, Canada

Shanta J. Persaud, London, UK

Nikolai Petrovsky, Canberra, Australia

John C. Pickup, London, UK

Jonathan Pinkney, Liverpool, UK

C.S. Pitchumoni, New York, USA

Toomas Podar, Tartu, Estonia

Paul Poirier, Québec, Canada

Julia M. Polak, London, UK

Michel Polak, Paris, France

G. Premalatha, Chennai, India

David Price, Swansea, UK

Jayaraj Rajagopal, Cambridge, MA, USA

Robert A. Rizza, Rochester, MN, USA

Christopher M. Ryan, Pittsburgh, PA, USA

Edmond A. Ryan, Edmonton, Canada

David Savage, Cambridge, UK

Desmond A. Schatz, Gainesville, FL, USA

Fraser W. Scott, Ottawa, Canada

A.M. James Shapiro, Edmonton, Canada

Graham R. Sharpe, Liverpool, UK

Ronald J. Sigal, Ottawa, Canada

Alan J. Sinclair, Coventry, UK

Jay S. Skyler, Miami, FL, USA

Gérard Slama, Paris, France

Tamar S. Smith, New York, USA

Tetsuya Taguchi, New York, USA

Robert B. Tattersall, Nottingham, UK

Nicholas Tentolouris, Athens, Greece

David R. Tomlinson, Manchester, UK

Peter C.Y. Tong, Shatin, Hong Kong

Hamish M.A. Towler, London, UK

Jaakko Tuomilehto, Helsinki, Finland

Martine Vaxillaire, Lille, France

Adrian Vella, Rochester, MN, USA

Giancarlo F. Viberti, London, UK

Tara M. Wallace, Oxford, UK

Maureen E. Wallymahmed, Liverpool, UK

Nils Welsh, Uppsala, Sweden

Morris F. White, Boston, MA, USA

John P.H. Wilding, Liverpool, UK

Gareth Williams, Bristol, UK

Stephen P. Wood, Southampton, UK

Hannele Yki-Järvinen, Helsinki, Finland

Ji-Won Yoon, Calgary, Canada

Matthew J. Young, Edinburgh, UK

Robert J. Young, Manchester, UK

Additional figures courtesy of:

1.4 Dr A Foulis, Glasgow, UK.
1.5a Professor R Bilous and Dr K White, University of Newcastle upon Tyne, UK.
1.7 Amos AF *et al. Diabet Med* 1997; **14**: S1–85.
2.1 The Wellcome Institute Library, London, UK.
2.2 Adapted from Papaspyros S. *The History of Diabetes Mellitus*, 2nd edn. Stuttgart: Thieme, 1964.
2.3 The Wellcome Institute Library, London, UK.
2.4 The Wellcome Institute Library, London, UK.
2.5 The Wellcome Institute Library, London, UK.
2.6 Bernard C. *Leçons de Physiologie Expérimentale Appliquées à la Médicine*. Paris: Baillière, 1855: 296–313.
2.9 The Wellcome Institute Library, London, UK.
2.10 The late Professor M Berger, Düsseldorf, Germany.
2.12 From the Thomas Fisher Rare Book Library, University of Toronto, Canada.
2.14 From the Thomas Fisher Rare Book Library, University of Toronto, Canada.
2.18 The Godfrey Argent Studio, London.
2.19 The Godfrey Argent Studio, London.
2.20 Diabetes UK.
3.1 Adapted from Expert Committee on the Diagnosis and Classification of Diabetes Mellitus. *Diabetes Care* 1997; **20**: 1183–97.

3.3 Adapted from Expert Committee on the Diagnosis and Classification of Diabetes Mellitus. *Diabetes Care* 1997; **20**: 1183–97.
3.6 Tattersall R, Gale E. *Am J Med* 1981; **70**:77–82.
3.7 Paisey RB. *Diabetologia* 1980; **19**: 31–4.
3.9 Harris MI *et al. Diabetes Care* 1992; **15**: 815–19.
3.10 Harris MI *et al. Diabetes Care* 1992; **15**: 815–19.
4.2 Marks HH, Krall LP. In: Marble A *et al.* eds. *Joslin's Diabetes Mellitus*, 12th edn. Philadelphia: Lea and Febiger, 1988: 209–54.
4.3 McNally PG *et al. Diabet Med* 1995; **12**: 961–6.
4.4 King H *et al. Diabetes Care* 1998; **21**: 1414–31.
4.7 Tuomilehto J *et al. N Engl J Med* 2001; **344**: 1343–50.
5.8b Orci L. *Diabetologia* 1974; **10**: 163–87.
6.4 Padaiga Z *et al. Diabet Med* 1999; **16**: 1–8.
6.5 Bodansky H J *et al. BMJ* 1992; **304**: 1020–2.
6.7 EURODIAB ACE Study Group. *Lancet* 2000; **355**: 873–6.
6.8 Dr A Foulis, Glasgow, UK.
6.10 Krischer JP *et al. J Clin Endocrinol Metab* 1993: **77**: 743–9.
6.20 Adapted from Scott FW *et al. Diabetes* 1997; **46**: 589–98.
6.21 Scott FLV. *Am J Clin Nutr* 1990; **51**: 489–91.
6.22 Sandler S. Abstracts of Uppsala Dissertations from the Faculty of Medicine, University of Uppsala, Sweden, 1983.

7.2　Adapted from King H *et al. Diabetes Care* 1993; **16**: 157–77.

7.4　Adapted from King H *et al. Diabetes Care* 1993; **16**: 157–77.

7.5　Harris MI *et al. Diabetes Care* 1998; **21**: 518–24.

7.6　King H *et al. Diabetes Care* 1998; **21**: 1414–31.

7.7　West K. *Epidemiology of Diabetes and its Vascular Lesions.* Elsevier, 1978.

7.8　Chan JM *et al. Diabetes Care* 1994: **17**: 961–9.

7.9　Jung RT. *Colour Atlas of Obesity.* London: Wolfe Medical Publications, 1990.

7.10　Dr H Lewis Jones, Liverpool, UK.

7.11　Pan DA *et al. Diabetes* 1997; **46**: 983–8.

7.13　Helmrich SB *et al. N Engl J Med* **325**: 147–52.

7.16　Hales CN, Barker DJP. *Diabetologia* 1992; **35**: 595–601.

7.17　UK Prospective Diabetes Study Group. *Diabetes* 1995; **44**:1249–58.

7.18　Polonsky KS *et al. N Engl J Med* 1998; **318**: 1231–9.

7.20　Dr GM Reaven, Stanford University, CA, USA.

8.2　Pearson ER *et al. Diabetes* 2001; **50**: S101–7, and Ellard S, Hattersley AT, unpublished.

8.5　Professor G Williams, University of Bristol, Bristol, UK.

8.8　Profesor JC Pickup, King's College, London, UK.

8.9　Professor G Williams, University of Bristol, Bristol, UK.

8.10　Moller DE, O'Rahilly S. In: Moller DE ed. *Insulin Resistance.* Chichester: John Wiley and Sons, 1993: 49–81.

8.11　Dr LJ Elsas, Emory University, Atlanta, GA, USA.

8.12　Dr AC McCuish, Dr JD Quin, Glasgow Royal Infirmary, Glasgow, UK.

8.14　Dr JS Flier, Beth Israel Hospital, Boston, MA, USA.

8.16　The late Professor M White, University of Hull, Hull, UK.

8.22　Professor S Bloom, Imperial College School of Medicine, London, UK.

9.5　Tattersall R, Gale E. *Am J Med* 1981; **70**:77–82.

9.9　Paisey RB. *Diabetologia* 1980; **19**: 31–4.

9.10　Data from Rohlfing CL *et al. Diabetes Care* 2002; **25**: 275–8.

9.11　Ashby JP, Frier BM. *Diabet Med* 1988; **5**: 118–21.

10.2　Owens DR *et al. Lancet* 2001; **358**: 739–46.

10.4　Eli Lilly and Co.

10.5　Dimitriadis GD, Gerich GE. *Diabetes Care* 1983; **6**: 374–7.

10.6　Brange J *et al. Diabetes Care* 1990; **13**: 923–54.

10.9　Lepore M *et al. Diabetes* 2000; **49**: 2142–8.

10.12　Dr G Gill, University of Liverpool, Liverpool, UK.

10.13　Reeves WG *et al. BMJ* 1980; **ii**: 1500–3.

10.18　Upper: Medtronic-MiniMed Inc, Northridge, CA, USA; Lower: Disetronic Medical Systems AG, Burgdorf, Switzerland.

10.20　Bode BW *et al. Diabetes Care* 1996; **19**: 324–7.

10.22　Medtronic-MiniMed Inc, Northridge, CA, USA.

10.23　Heinemann L *et al. Diabet Med* 1997; **14**: 63–72.

11.2　Heilbronn LK *et al. Diabetes Care* 1999; **22**: 889–95.

11.3　Hollander PA *et al. Diabetes Care* 1998; **21**: 1288–94.

11.6　Al-Delaimy WK *et al. Diabetes Care* 2001; **24**: 2043–8.

11.8　UKPDS Group. *Lancet* 1998; **352**: 837–54.

11.16　Bailey CJ. *Pharm Sci* 2000; **21**: 259–65.

12.9　Professor G. Williams, University of Bristol, Bristol, UK.

12.10　Professor G. Williams, University of Bristol, Bristol, UK.

13.3　Diabetes Control and Complications Trial. *N Engl J Med* 1993; **329**: 977–86.

13.8　Boli GB *et al. Diabetes* 1983; **32**: 134–41.

13.9　Pramming S *et al. Diabet Med* 1991; **8**: 217–27.

14.1　Pirart J. *Diabetes Care* 1978; **1**: 168–88, 262–61.

14.2　Klein R *et al. Ann Intern Med* 1996; **124**: 90–6.

14.3　Diabetes Control and Complications Trial. *N Engl J Med* 1993; **329**: 977–86.

14.4　Diabetes Control and Complications Trial. *N Engl J Med* 1993; **329**: 977–86.

14.5　UKPDS Group. *Lancet* 1998; **352**: 837–54.

14.6　UKPDS Group. *BMJ* 1998; **317**: 703–13.

14.7　Diabetes Control and Complications Trial/Epidemiology of Diabetes Interventions and Complications Research Group. *N Engl J Med* 2000; **342**; 381–9.

14.8　Khaw K *et al. BMJ* 2001; **322**: 15–18.

15.13　Dr PJ Barry, Royal Victoria Eye and Ear Hospital, Belfast, UK.

16.1　Professor R Bilous and Dr K White, University of Newcastle upon Tyne, UK.

16.2　Professor R Bilous and Dr K White, University of Newcastle upon Tyne, UK.

16.4　Borch-Johnsen K *et al. Diabetologia* 1989; **28**: 590–6.

16.5　Toumilehto J *et al. Diabetologia* 1998; **41**: 784–90.

16.6　Norgaard K *et al. Diabetologia* 1990; **33**: 407–10.

16.10　Anon. *Diabetes* 1996; **45**: 1289–98.

16.11　ACE Inhibitors in Diabetic Nephropathy Trialist Group. *Ann Intern Med* 2001; **134**: 370–9.

16.12　Viberti GC *et al. Lancet* 1982; **i**: 1430–2.

16.14　Quinn M *et al. Diabetologia* 1996; **39**: 940–5.

16.15　Barzilay J *et al. Kidney Int* 1992; **41**: 723–30.

16.17　Jones RH *et al. Lancet* 1979; **i**: 1105–6.

16.18 Parving H-H *et al. BMJ* 1987; **294**: 1443–7.
17.4 Dr G Gill, University of Liverpool, Liverpool, UK.
17.9 Professor G Williams, University of Bristol, Bristol, UK.
17.13 Diabetes Control and Complications Trial Research Group. *Ann Intern Med* 1995; **122**: 566–8.
18.19 Pyorala K *et al. Diabetes Care* 1997; **20**: 614–20.
19.5 Krolewski AS *et al. Am J Med* 1985; **78**: 785–94.
19.7 UKPDS Group. *BMJ* 1998; **317**: 703–13.
20.1 Haffner SM *et al. N Engl J Med* 1998; **339**: 229–34.
20.5 Data from Stammler J *et al. Diabetes Care* 1993; **16**: 434–44.
20.6 Data from Jarrett RJ, Shipley MJ. *Diabetologia* 1988; **31**: 737–40.
20.10 Herlitz J *et al. Acta Med Scand* 1988; **224**: 31–8.
20.11 Data from Pyörälä K *et al. Diabet Metab Rev* 1987; **3**: 463–542.
20.12 Data from Pyörälä K *et al. Diabet Metab Rev* 1987; **3**: 463–542.
20.15 Malmberg K *et al. J Am Coll Cardiol* 1995; **26**: 57–65.
21.5 Dr G Gill, University of Liverpool, Liverpool, UK.
21.8 Professor G Williams, University of Bristol, Bristol, UK.
21.11 Professor G Williams, University of Bristol, Bristol, UK.
21.17 Novartis Ltd.
22.1 Bancroft J. *Human Sexuality and its Problems*. Edinburgh: Churchill Livingstone, 1989.
22.15 Lawrensen RA *et al. Diabet Med* 1999; **16**: 395–9.
22.17 Løkkegaard E *et al. BMJ* 2003; **326**: 426–8.
23.2 Rayner C *et al. Diabetes Care* 2001; **24**: 371–81.
23.3 Scharcz E *et al. Diabet Med* 1993; **10**: 660–3.
23.4 Horowitz M *et al. J Gastroenterol Hepatol* 1998; **13**: S239–45.
23.5 Adapted from Holloway RH *et al. Am J Gastroenterol* 1999; **94**: 3150–7.

24.1 Professor J Verbov, University of Liverpool, Liverpool, UK.
24.6 Dr G Gill, University of Liverpool, Liverpool, UK.
24.8 Dr S Mendelsohn, Countess of Chester Hospital, Chester, UK.
24.12 Dr S Mendelsohn, Countess of Chester Hospital, Chester, UK.
24.19 Professor JC Pickup, King's College, London, UK.
25.2 Anderson RJ *et al. Diabetes Care* 2001; **24**: 1069–78.
25.5 Ryan C *et al. Pediatrics* 1985; **75**: 921–7.
26.1 Devlin JT *et al. Diabetes* 1987; **36**; 434–9.
26.3 Moy CS *et al. Am J Epidemiol* 1993; **137**: 74–81.
26.10 Dr I MacFarlane Walton Hospital, Liverpool, UK.
26.11 Professor G Williams, University of Bristol, Bristol, UK.
26.12 Rupp ME. *N Engl J Med* 1995; **333**: 564.
27.3 Dr I MacFarlane, Walton Hospital, Liverpool, UK.
27.4 Professor C Lowy, St Thomas' Hospital, London, UK.
28.1 Green A *et al. Lancet* 2000; **355**: 873–6.
28.6 Mortensen HB *et al. Diabetes Care* 1997; **20**: 714–20.
29.1 Harris MI *et al. Diabetes Care* 1998; **21**: 518–24.
30.3 Dr D Flanagan, Addenbrooke's Hospital, Cambridge, UK.
30.4 Waclawski ER. *Diabet Med* 1989; **6**: 16–19.
30.6 Suarez L, Barrett-Connor E. *Am J Epidemiol* 1984; **120**: 670–5.
31.1 Adapted from Knight AH. In: *Textbook of Diabetes*, 2nd edn. Oxford: Blackwell Science, 1997: 79.1–9.
31.3 Miller LV, Goldstein J. *N Engl J Med* 1972; **286**: 1388–91.
32.1 International Pancreas Transplant Registry.
32.2 Dr S Barlett, University of Maryland, MD, USA.

INDEX

Regranex 201
regulated pathway of insulin secretion 32
renal threshold 17
renal transplantation 162
repaglinide 111, 114
respiratory distress syndrome
    adult 123
    neonatal 239
respiratory tract infections 234
restless legs 168
retinal detachment 148
retinal photocoagulation 179
retinoid X receptor 174
retrovirus-like particles 48
revascularization 194
rhinocerebral mucormycosis 234
Rhizopus spp. 234
Rollo, John 7
rosiglitazone 111, 115
rosuvastatin 173
Rothera's test 90

S

Sanger, Frederick 12
Scandinavian Simvastatin Survival Study
    174
Scott, Ernest 9
screening 18–19
self-monitoring 85
sertraline 227
serum cholesterol 171
sexual problems 203–9
    in men 204–7
    in women 208–9
shin spots 218
sialic acid 68
sibutramine 108, 111
sildenafil (Viagra) 207
simvastatin 173
skin and connective tissue disorders
    217–22
    acanthosis nigricans 76, 220
    cheiroarthropathy 219
    diabetic bullae 221
    diabetic dermopathy 218
    Dupuytren's contracture 220
    erythema multiforme 222
    frozen shoulder 220
    insulin-induced lipoatrophy 222
    lipohypertrophy 99, 222
    necrobiosis lipoidica diabeticorum
        218–19
    paronychia 221
    Stevens–Johnson syndrome 222
    tinea manus 221
    trigger finger 220
    see also individual conditions
smoking 110, 256
somatostatin 29
sorbitol 138
split proinsulins 32
Staphylococcus aureus 234

statins 173–4
stem-cell therapy 265–6
Stevens–Johnson syndrome 222
Streptococcus spp. 234
streptozocin 52
stroke 191
substance P 168s
sulphonylureas 33, 111, 112–14
superoxide 142
surgery 235–6
Susruta 6
syndrome X 66, 170, 176, 189
systemic lupus erythematosus 77

T

telmisartan 181
thiazolidinediones 111, 115
Thompson, Leonard 11
'thrifty phenotype' hypothesis 63
thromboembolism 123
tinea manus 221
tirofiban 192
tolazamide 111, 113
tolbutamide 111, 113
trandolapril 180
transforming growth factor-β_1 159
transient ischaemic attacks 191
travel 257
tricyclic antidepressants 168
trigger finger 220
triglyceride 170
troglitazone 115
truncal radiculopathy 167
tumour necrosis factor 60
Turner, Robert 12
type 1 diabetes 2, 20, 39–53
    aetiology 40
    autoimmune 44–5
    blood lipid abnormalities 171
    characteristics 21
    environmental influences 41–3, 48
    familial clustering 42
    frequency 44
    genetic susceptibility 46–7
    hypertension 178
    management 93–105
    prevalence 41–3
        geographical 41–3
        seasonal variation in 42
    virus-related 48–9
type 2 diabetes 2, 3, 20, 55–69
    β-cell function 63–4
    blood lipid abnormalities 170
    characteristics 21
    in children 247
    genetic defect in 62
    genetic predisposition 61–2
    hypertension 176–7
    insulin resistance 60, 65–6
    insulin secretion 32
    and intrauterine/neonatal nutrition
        63

and lack of exercise 61
management 107–16
    anti-obesity drugs 108
    diet 109
    exercise 110
    oral hypoglycaemics 110–16
    stopping smoking 110
    weight loss 108
and pancreatic carcinoma 76
pregnancy 242
prevalence 26, 56–8
    age-related 58
    geographical 56–7
risk factors 56
type A insulin resistance 76
type B insulin resistance 77

U

UK National Guidelines on Screening for
    Diabetic Retinopathy 144
UK Prospective Diabetes Study (UKPDS)
    12, 89, 136, 158, 188
ulnar nerve compression 166
ultralente insulin 97
uric acid 189
urinary albumin excretion 157
urinary tract infections 233
urine glucose testing 86
urine ketone testing 90
urine, sugar in *see* glycosuria
urine testing strips 86

V

valproate 168
valsartan 181
vascular cell adhesion molecule-1 *see*
    VCAM-1
vascular endothelial growth factor 140,
    159
vasoactive intestinal peptide 29
VCAM-1 140, 188, 189
verapamil 181
very-low-density lipoprotein 66, 170
Viagra 207
viruses in type 1 diabetes 48–9
vitamin B$_{12}$ deficiency 168
vitiligo 77
vitreoretinal surgery 150
Vivoderm Autograft System 201
von Mering, Joseph 8

W

wheat gluten, as cause of diabetes 50
Willis, Thomas 6
Wisconsin Epidemiologic Study of Diabetic
    Retinopathy 134
Wolfram syndrome 79, 244
World Health Organization 14

Z

Zuelzer, George 9